COPI

Examines the na
how it affects s

Coping with
BULIMIA
THE BINGE-PURGE SYNDROME

Barbara French

Thorsons
An Imprint of HarperCollins*Publishers*

Thorsons
An Imprint of HarperCollins*Publishers*
77–85 Fulham Palace Road,
Hammersmith, London W6 8JB
1160 Battery Street,
San Francisco, California 94111–1213

Published by Thorsons 1987
This edition 1994
1   3   5   7   9   10   8   6   4   2

A catalogue record for this book
is available from the British Library

ISBN 0 7225 2944 9

Printed and bound by
HarperCollins Manufacturing, Glasgow

ACKNOWLEDGEMENTS

I am deeply grateful to all the women who so willingly and bravely shared their innermost thoughts, feelings and experiences of bulimia with me. They contributed a great deal to the creation of the book and motivated me to keep working on it when I was tempted to give up.

I would also like to thank everyone who was involved in the Edinburgh Eating Disorder Group in 1984 and 1985; Dr Christopher Freeman, who realized the need for self-help information for bulimia sufferers long before I did; and Dr Jane Turnbull, Fiona Barry, Annette Annandale and Mike Henderson for their professional opinions, advice and encouragement. I would also like to acknowledge my indebtedness to Dr Alex Crawford for helping me to clarify a number of points concerning problem drinking.

I am also grateful to Marie Mercer, Margaret Grainger and Kerry McCrindle for letting me lean on their secretarial skills, and to my father for reading early drafts of the manuscript and making valuable suggestions for its improvement.

My special thanks are reserved for my children, William and Katherine, who at the tender ages of four and two, did all that they could to give me the time and the space I needed to write the book.

DEDICATION

For Bill, whose loyalty, love and understanding carried
me through days of darkness and self doubt.

CONTENTS

FOREWORD

Over the past fifteen to twenty years, bulimia has become the most common type of eating problem that is referred to psychiatrists and psychologists for treatment. Studies in the United Kingdom and America have shown that between 1 and 2 percent of women in general, and between 4 and 5 percent of the late adolescent and young female population suffer from this syndrome. This means that there may be more than half a million women with bulimia in the United Kingdom. Occasional episodes of bingeing and vomiting are probably much more common than this. One study has shown that up to 15 percent of women may binge and/or vomit from time to time. Of course, not all women who binge and vomit want or even need psychological treatment. Some may accept it as an inevitable consequence of their dieting. Others may vomit occasionally to avoid absorbing large amounts of calories after a big meal. At the other end of the spectrum, bulimia in its most severe form is an extremely distressing and potentially life-threatening condition, which can totally dominate a woman's life. Many sufferers feel very ashamed and guilty about their behaviour, and most are reluctant to discuss it with their general practitioner. In fact, they often do not discuss it with anyone so that their behaviour and consequent suffering remain secret.

Because of the large number of sufferers and the secret nature of the problem, there is no way that existing health service resources can treat everyone. Self-help is therefore a particularly important and valuable approach.

This book presents a balanced and sensible self-help programme for bulimia. It is particularly important that it is written by a woman, since nearly all those with bulimia are women, and that it is written by someone who has experienced the syndrome herself. Although a number of other self-help books deal with eating disorders, most of them concentrate on anorexia nervosa rather than bulimia. Clearly, there are important links between the two conditions, but there are also many important differences. Only a minority of women who have bulimia have a previous history of anorexia nervosa. Most women who start binge-eating have never been markedly underweight. One major difference between the two syndromes is that it is almost impossible to keep anorexia nervosa a secret. The mere fact that the sufferer looks so thin, drawn and haggard is a very public statement that she is ill, and this immediately attracts attention and concern. Sometimes that is what the sufferer wants, but not always. In contrast, women with bulimia are able to keep their problem concealed and may suffer privately for many years, desperately wanting help but too ashamed to approach anyone for it.

The few books that are available on bulimia tend to promote one particular viewpoint of the disorder. This book looks at the problem from many angles and will be a great help to anyone who suffers from bulimia as well as to relatives and friends of sufferers. There is a very comprehensive section on the main signs and symptoms of the disorder and on the medical and physical consequences of repeated bingeing and vomiting. The second half of the book contains a detailed self-help programme, illustrated with clinical examples. There is also guidance on how to seek help from others.

Finally, bulimia is a problem that tends to recur. When you have had a habit for many years it is not too difficult to slip back into old ways at times of stress or unhappiness, even after successful treatment. Such people may be reluctant to go and seek help again, so knowing how to help themselves is particularly important.

Dr Christopher Freeman
Consultant Psychiatrist

April 1986

INTRODUCTION

My life revolves around mindlessly stuffing myself with whole
loaves of bread, pots of jam, platefuls of biscuits and litres of
lemonade. If I have no money, anything lying around the
kitchen will do.

The more I eat, the worse I feel, the worse I feel, the more I
stuff myself, until I'm physically bloated and stoned out of my
mind.

I've become a victim of my obsession. It's like being locked
on a treadmill of self-destruction, and no matter what I eat, I'm
making myself sick shortly afterwards.

These comments describe the frenzied pattern of behaviour
which traps victims of bulimia, or the binge-purge
syndrome. Food is a well-recognized source of comfort and
enjoyment, as well as being of nutritional value, and many
people turn to eating for its pacifying effects during
moments of stress, boredom or loneliness. But sufferers of
bulimia get little pleasure from food. Constant thoughts
about their diet, weight, and body shape generate great
tension. Uncontrollable urges to eat and then rid
themselves (by self-induced vomiting, laxative abuse or
both) of the large amounts of food taken, wreak havoc with
their physical and emotional well-being and often take a
heavy financial toll.

This book has been written for bulimia sufferers and for
relatives and friends who want to know more about this
condition. Despite the potentially crippling effects of the
disorder, public knowledge remains scanty. Women who
embark on the binge-purge cycle as a means of controlling
their weight often do not realize the hazards involved.
What may have seemed the perfect solution to the dietary

dilemma of wanting to eat but not gain weight can rapidly become a nightmarish existence of wild excesses and intolerable restrictions, within which sufferers feel bewildered and cornered. Once this destructive lifestyle is established, many despair of ever being able to piece together their fragmented lives, and so they become deeply depressed.

The aim of this book is to provide knowledge and insight into the origins and symptoms of bulimia. It is hoped that, armed with a fuller understanding of the condition, sufferers will be able to unravel some of the causes of their own eating problems, and that they will feel strengthened and encouraged in their struggle to 'climb out of the rut'. Those who feel hopelessly isolated and locked within this condition may be comforted and reassured to know that they are not alone. Attitudes and thoughts relating to daily situations have been taken from interviews to illustrate the viewpoints and feelings which women with bulimia often share. It is hoped that these will dispel the fears experienced by so many sufferers that they are bizarre freaks.

Although the book is aimed primarily at sufferers and their families, it is hoped that other readers will also find the information enlightening. Bulimia is very much a hidden problem. Interest and concern is occasionally, and rather sensationally, generated by the media, but there is an acute need for a greater general awareness of the problem and more open recognition of its existence. Only then will some of the prejudice and shame attached to the condition be set aside, so that victims feel confident enough to obtain the support they so badly need from family, friends and society.

The second half of the book addresses sufferers personally. It contains a wide range of self-help strategies and ideas for overcoming bulimia which it is hoped will act as useful supplements to professional help. It also contains an outline of treatment currently available from the National Health Service, independent counselling services and self-help groups.

Note: Although men also suffer from bulimia, this is less common, so for the sake of simplicity sufferers have been referred to as 'she' throughout the text.

PART 1.

UNDERSTANDING BULIMIA

1.

WHAT IS BULIMIA?

Bulimia is an eating disorder characterized by uncontrollable bouts of over-eating followed by self-induced vomiting and/or laxative abuse to get rid of the food.

A variety of other names have been coined to describe this condition including, bulimarexia, the 'binge-purge cycle', the 'stuffing syndrome', and the 'dietary chaos syndrome'. Hilde Bruch, an American authority on eating disorders, applied the term 'fat/thin people' to those with symptoms of bulimia. She observed that some people who are overweight (which many sufferers of bulimia are, before they develop the condition) and who subsequently succeed in becoming thin 'still resemble fat people with all their unresolved conflicts and exaggerated expectations, only they no longer show their fat'. Although these people may initially feel pleased because they have lost weight, they still have unresolved anxieties, poor self-esteem, or confusion about how they want their lives to go. Rather than tackling these separately, they regard their physical appearance as the cause of all their problems. They believe that by controlling their weight they will gain control of their lives. Inevitably, losing weight fails to produce the desired confidence, success and happiness which they seek, but many sufferers are unable to appreciate that weight control is not the answer. They may slide into a condition of starving to lose yet more weight, and bingeing when cravings for food overcome them. They then need to purge themselves to avoid putting on weight and so the cycle is established.

2.

HOW COMMON IS BULIMIA?

Bulimia is associated in many people's minds with anorexia nervosa. Indeed, it has been recognized for some time that some anorexics suffer from bulimia as a second stage of their disorder. There have been suggestions in various publications that bulimia is not a common problem. Medical papers have described it as 'an ominous variant of anorexia nervosa'.[1] When the model Pauline Seaward died as the result of an enormous binge following a three-day fast, newspapers said that she suffered from 'a rare and advanced form of the slimmers' disease anorexia nervosa'.

In recent years, however, it has been realized that bulimia is a separate condition, although it can occur as a result of other eating disorders. It also affects far more people than was originally thought, and these are not necessarily women with a history of eating disorders. Studies have shown that one in twenty–five first year female students from Edinburgh University suffered from symptoms of bulimia in 1983, and successive Edinburgh surveys have repeatedly confirmed this figure. Studies of female college students in America[2] and Australia[3] have shown roughly one in ten to fulfill strict criteria for the bulimia syndrome[4]. The results of further research are awaited, but it seems probable that as bulimia is such a guilt-ridden and secretive condition the true incidence could be even higher. Earlier studies of eating behaviour show that disordered and irregular eating patterns do seem to be remarkably common. For example, in 1981 a survey of female American college students[5] showed that up to one in three binged and one in eight vomited food.

Bulimia nervosa and anorexia nervosa

Approximately 40–50 percent of people who suffer from anorexia will develop bulimia. Although there are similarities between the two conditions, such as attitudes concerning control of food intake and the overwhelming fear of fatness, each disorder has its distinguishing features. These are summarized in the table below.

Table 1 Characteristics of Bulimia and Anorexia

Characteristic	Bulimia	Anorexia
Background	Mixed social strata	Largely middle class
Age of onset	The majority of cases occur between the ages of 16 and 45, usually at 20–25	Usually during teenage years
Personality	Extrovert, articulate, socially competent, sexually experienced	More introverted, tends to depend on family and to be sexually inexperienced
Eating habits	Binge/purge cycles; sufferer turns to food in stress; feels she has lost control of eating	Binge/purge far less frequent; sufferer turns away from food in stress; rigid control of diet
Appearance	Usually within the normal range for height and weight	Very thin, often emaciated
Attitudes to body weight and shape	Weight may be a less important consideration than binge/purge cycles	Body weight is all-absorbing

Characteristic	Bulimia	Anorexia
Physiological effects	Disturbed menstruation caused by stress and chaotic eating; secondary effects of vomiting	Menstruation ceases. Stigmata of starvation
Attitudes to eating problem	Aware of problem and disturbed by it – this may eventually prompt them to seek and accept help.	Adamant refusal to accept that anything is wrong
Depression	May be very severe; sufferer is overwhelmed by feelings of self-disgust and anger at losing control	May be less severe; keeping her weight under control is a constant spur and reward to the sufferer's morale

Bulimia in Men

Men can suffer from bulimia, but it does not seem to be a common occurrence. In the 1983 Edinburgh Student Survey into bulimia, for example, 1,500 male and female students took part and only one male sufferer came to light. In the same year a study of 303 Australian university students was carried out[6]. 97 males and 206 females participated and the only sufferers identified were women.

We do not know why eating disorders are largely restricted to women. One reason may be that the factors which are thought to influence the development of bulimia apply far more directly to women than to men. These are discussed in chapter 4, 'Risk Factors'.

Another clue may lie in the different ideas men and women have about their shape. Many normal women tend to over-estimate their size, while those with bulimia and anorexia see themselves as bloated and fat in the extreme.

Male victims of anorexia, however, seem able to retain a more realistic mental picture of themselves. Men do not seem to have the same pre-occupation with the attractiveness of being thin that women do. Although they may suffer the same loss of self-esteem and feelings of worthlessness, they are less likely to look to dieting as a means of restoring their self-confidence and of making them more attractive to women. Thus they avoid one of the major triggering factors for the development of bulimia, which is ravenous hunger as a result of strict dieting.

Examples of male bulimia victims are athletes, jockeys and dancers, who probably started dieting because of their work rather than worries about their appearance.

[1] Russell, G.F.M. (1979). *Bulimia Nervosa: An ominous variant of Anorexia Nervosa.* Psychological Medicine, 9, pp.429–448.

[2] Collins, M., Kreisberg, J., Pertschuk, M. and Fager, S. (1982). *Bulimia in college women. Prevalence and psychopathology.* Journal of Adolescent Health Care, 3.144.

[3] Touyz, S. and Ivison, D. (1983). *Bulimia: A survey of an Australian University Population.* Proceedings of the eighteenth Annual Conference of the Psychological Society, Sydney, p.99.

[4] People are considered to have the bulimia syndrome if they fulfill criteria defined by the Diagnostic and Statistical Manual of Mental Disorders, 3rd Edition (DSM III). *See* Table 2 below.

[5] Halmi, K.A., Falk, J.R. and Schwartz, E. (1981). *Binge eating and vomiting: A survey of a college population.* Psychological Medicine, 11. 697–706.

[6] Touyz, S. and Ivison, D. (1983).

Table 2   DSM III Diagnostic Criteria for Bulimia

A Recurrent episodes of binge-eating (rapid consumption of a large amount of food in a discrete period of time, usually less than two hours).

B At least three of the following:
  (i) consumption of high-caloric, easily ingested food during a binge
  (ii) inconspicuous eating during a binge
  (iii) termination of such eating episodes for abdominal pain, sleep, social interruption, or self-induced vomiting
  (iv) repeated attempts to lose weight by severely restrictive diets, self-induced vomiting, or use of cathartics or diuretics
  (v) frequent weight fluctuations greater than 10 pounds due to alternating binges and fasts.

C Awareness that the eating pattern is abnormal and fear of not being able to stop eating voluntarily.

D Depressed mood and self-deprecating thoughts following eating binges.

E The bulimic episodes are not due to anorexia nervosa or any known physical disorder.

3.

GENERAL CHARACTERISTICS

People who suffer from bulimia in later life were often quiet and well-behaved children who were always good and obedient. Fear of rejection or of parental disapproval may have made them anxious to please by being grown-up and independent at a young age. As adolescents they may have been easy-going, passive and eager to win the approval of their family and friends:

> I can't remember a time in my childhood when I really misbehaved. I was always trying to be Little Miss Likeable, wanting pats on the back from everyone and continually shifting my viewpoint to accommodate the opinions of others.

> My parents took great pride in telling others how I never gave them any trouble. My mother spoke about me as her 'little angel'. In actual fact I saw myself as something of a stuffed dummy. I had no views on anything... no sense of self. I was a bit like a chameleon, always changing my colours so that I harmonized with what everyone else thought or wanted to do.

They may have gained weight during puberty, as many girls do, and then developed anxieties about their size or shape because it was fashionable to be slim. A teasing or casual comment about their appearance may have prompted them to lose weight by dieting. What began as a period of strict dieting then led on to a more long-term eating problem.

Appearances
Unlike anorexics, bulimia sufferers are not easy to spot because they seem to eat normally when they are with other people, most of them are the normal weight for their

age and height, and they go on their eating binges in private. In fact, many sufferers find that their weight fluctuates quite a bit because of their chaotic eating, but these changes often happen over a very short space of time, and they tend to choose clothes that hide the facts from others.

One reason the condition tends to be so puzzling and difficult for others to understand is that sufferers frequently appear cheery, full of life, and self-assured. Many are talented, intelligent and attractive, but their appearance belies their fragile self-esteem and immense inner distress at being so out of control about food.

> I suppose I looked like one of those fortunate people who has everything going for them – a nice place to live, a job with good prospects, and a kind and attentive boyfriend. I had no reason to be unhappy, except that always having to keep my distance from people in case they discovered my awful secret, made me miserable and depressed. Deep down, I hated myself such a lot and felt unworthy of anyone's love.

As sufferers retreat further into their private world of bingeing and purging, their sense of isolation grows and they fear that one day they will be 'found out'.

> I lived in mortal fear that this disgusting habit of mine would be discovered. Life became a game of 'cat and mouse' between me and my boyfriend. He often wondered why I spent so long closeted behind locked bathroom doors, supposedly having a bath, washing my hair and so on. When he got home he'd be baffled at the urgency with which I'd despatch him to the shops for some trivial item. Usually it was so that I could either finish a binge or make myself sick without the strain of having to hide what I was doing from him.

The stress which results from having to cover their tracks may be immense. Sometimes it causes even more bingeing, because eating is the one thing which relieves their tension.

Most sufferers are aware that their eating is abnormal, but shame, guilt and self disgust may make them initially reluctant to admit the problem to themselves, sometimes for years, let alone confide in anyone else about it. Coming to terms with the fact that they have a problem can be a traumatic experience and it may take years to overcome.

I'd turned a blind eye to the fact that anything was wrong for four years. It was a painful time of waking up and realizing the terrible truth–I was in one hell of a mess.

However, with the right help and support, many sufferers come to feel relieved that they no longer have to keep their condition a fearfully guarded secret.

Self-dislike and criticism

Many women worry about their figures at some stage in their lives. These are very different worries from the ingrained and unremitting self-doubts of women with bulimia. They tend to be very vulnerable to the barrage of propaganda about the importance of being slim and healthy and often have unrealistic expectations about what slimness might achieve for them. Many believe that they will only be happy and lovable if they look slim and beautiful. Areas of the body about which they are particularly sensitive include the thighs, bottom, face, legs and stomach, and many are unable to look at their reflection without thinking disparaging thoughts.

> I know I'm slim, but I'm never slim enough. The proportions of my body are never right. Never a day goes by when I don't look in the mirror and wonder how I might get rid of all these ugly pounds. They fill me with self-hatred. My thighs are too fat, my hips are so hefty, my face is too round, and so on. Sometimes I think the only thing that will make me happy would be a total body transplant.

Most sufferers are anxious to keep their weight at a certain point. They strive for an 'ideal' level which, although within the normal range according to height and weight tables, is usually towards the low end of this range and often a considerable underestimate for their actual physique. They may see thinness as the only goal in life which is socially valued and which will earn them respect.

> I dread the thought of becoming fat because I think I would lose respect. People would treat me with contempt and see that I have no control. My size would be visible proof of my pathetic, muddled, greedy, self indulgent nature.

Those who reach, and want to remain, at an unnaturally low weight may see no option to vomiting up the food. This is an effective way of becoming slim and staying that way, but nutritional deficiencies resulting from the restricted food intake and purging spark off intense cravings for food.

As the bingeing and purging becomes more frequent, sufferers often have difficulty in identifying sensations of hunger and lose all sense of what constitutes a normal amount of food. They soon get into the habit of overeating and then purging themselves by self-induced vomiting or by laxative abuse.

> My day centred around binge after binge interspersed with putting my fingers down my throat to make myself sick. Eating and vomiting became inseparable acts.

Attempts to alter their figure may not stop at dieting and purging. Some become very active, and daily jogging, dancing, swimming, 'working out' in a gym or doing aerobics may become part of their compensatory mechanism for losing weight.

> I put myself through unremitting agony trying to virtually beat my body into a better shape. I'd gallop up every flight of stairs I could find, stay awake until the small hours of the morning in the belief that I was burning up extra calories, spend several hours a day either jogging or swimming, and developed the strange idea that by wrapping my legs in polythene bin liners I would be able to sweat off fat.

Strained relationships and underlying problems

Personal anxieties and deeply ingrained self-doubts tend to make it difficult for bulimia sufferers to form close relationships with other people. They may also feel envious and slightly hostile to women whom they think have better figures:

> Jane was a good friend of mine, but the fact that she appeared to have an appetite like a horse, and could eat as much 'junk' food as she liked, without it ever showing, annoyed me intensely. She was sickeningly slinky.

Erratic mood swings caused by their chaotic eating pattern can make sufferers extremely difficult to live with.

> No-one could stand being with me for more than a couple of months. One moment I'd be lively and loving, the next I'd become this desperate person... self-centred and mean-

minded. My mood swings were all tied up with my eating
problem. Sometimes I felt as if I had a double personality.

I'd pick fights about nothing and fly off the handle at the
tiniest irritation. My aggression would drive people away, and
I suppose this was what I wanted – so that I could binge in
privacy.

Stormy relationships which ultimately break down are not
uncommon. Some people drive themselves deeper into
their bingeing/purging ritual when a relationship does not
work out. They see this as a way of insulating themselves
from personal involvements which they fear may become
emotionally or sexually demanding. A few sufferers are
described as promiscuous. Explanations for this have been
put forward by some professionals who, like Sigmund
Freud, are much concerned with the sexual significance of
various conditions. They relate over-eating to sexual hang-
ups of one sort or another and maintain that whilst binge-
eating serves to dampen down sexual feelings for some
women, for others it is a substitute for erotic gratification.
The physical act of eating, consisting of desire with
salivation, is thought by some pyschiatrists to resemble that
of sexual union. In her book *Night Thoughts* (Weidenfeld
and Nicolson, 1982), the American sex therapist Avodah
Offit describes this resemblance as the excitement of
tasting, chewing and the orgasmic contraction of
swallowing... Thus it has been suggested that individuals
who are unable to express or admit to having sexual desires,
or who reject their femininity, may turn to eating for erotic
pleasure. With regard to the promiscuous sufferer, her
'voracious appetite' may be seen as a reflection of her
insatiable sexual 'hunger', which she attempts to either curb
or satisfy through bingeing. Such people also have an ever-
changing cast of partners and, not surprisingly, are unable
to form close, meaningful relationships.

Another side to the 'psycho-sexual' theory on bulimia is
that women binge-eat as a result of over-identifying with
traditional feminine values, rather than rejecting them.
They are said to have a deep-seated commitment to the
popular image of femininity – the role of dependent
mistress, accommodating wife, sacrificial mother, nurse and
so on – and are anxious because they may not be living up
to their own and society's expectations of them. Such fears

generate a sense of failure, guilt, and frustration which they attempt to escape from.

Psycho-sexual interpretations of bulimia often annoy sufferers. They see no connection between them and their own situation, and refuse to take them seriously. They do not feel that bulimia victims are any more promiscuous than anyone else. Indeed, a study of 150 sufferers in Edinburgh would seem to bear this out, and those who are promiscuous cannot necessarily relate their behaviour to their bulimia. Sufferers who also have problems with alcohol, for example, may have become promiscuous because their sexual inhibitions are reduced by the effects of alcohol rather than because of an insatiable sex drive.

Many sufferers do not connect bingeing with their sex lives at all. Others only look at the effect of purging in this light because this is what makes them feel slimmer and therefore more attractive and desirable.

The truth is that there is no such thing as a typical 'bulimic'. Professionals are fond of putting people into tidy descriptive slots, but to suggest that bulimia sufferers in general are 'driven' by underlying sexual difficulties and/or gender role anxieties overlooks the fact that each individual is a unique blend of emotions. One person's unconscious motives, sexual or otherwise, will never be exactly the same as someone else's.

> Bingeing as a means of denying my sexuality never featured in my memory bank. If there was any relationship between by bulimia and my sex life, I would say it was more to do with the getting rid of the food. If I was full I'd feel ugly, and irritable, and couldn't bear anyone to touch me. If I'd managed to get rid of what I'd eaten I'd feel slim, desirable, and affectionate.

Depression, feelings of worthlessness and a sense of life being dull and meaningless may account for the food–orientated and flighty lifestyle of some individuals, whilst others are simply looking for an assurance from someone that they are needed, loved and appreciated.

> I've always wanted warmth and affection and I am a fairly demonstrative sort of person, but I wouldn't consider myself a scarlet woman with an unquenchable sex drive. Looking back, I can see that a simple cuddle would have helped to solve a lot of my problems. I wanted to feel safe, to know that someone cared about me, otherwise what was the point of existing?

I've had an all preoccupying desire for affection and approval for as long as I can remember. My therapist attributes this to an insecure childhood, which I suppose figures. My father was in the forces, so we did a lot of globe-trotting, and I never really had the opportunity to grow any roots or to make close friends. My efforts to win approval and reassure myself that I was lovable started out innocently enough, but became horribly complicated. The men I became involved with didn't seem to know that women need a bit of romance and appreciation, sexual qualities aside, before slipping in between the sheets.

Patterns of behaviour

Apart from a preoccupation with their appearance, many sufferers engage in repetitive rituals centred around their fears of gaining weight. These may include assessing themselves in the mirror several times a day, trying on their entire wardrobe regularly to make sure all their clothes fit in a certain way, feeling 'ruled' by the scales to the extent that they weigh themselves several times a day, and preparing, cooking, or eating food in a particular manner.

I would scrutinize every morsel of food for fat globules. I also took great care never to touch anything that had been near a pan of frying food in case it was contaminated with splattered fat. Anything remotely greasy had to be blotted between two sheets of kitchen paper to soak up the fat, and even then I'd have reservations about eating it.

Perfectionism

Striving for perfectionism is a characteristic trait amongst sufferers. Although many are academically bright, conscientious and intelligent, they still worry that they are not doing well enough, either in their work or in terms of being 'good enough' for other people.

I'm a complete workaholic, and want everything I do to be exactly right. If it's not, and it often isn't, I automatically start to see myself as an incompetent blockhead. I'll spend days thinking about what a failure I am, and wonder what the point is of trying anything.

Such high expectations and harsh self-judgement undermine their self-esteem and take away all sense of their personal achievement so that they may be unable to appreciate anything positive about themselves. Instead they become obsessed with their own exaggerated or imagined short comings.

> I'm continually comparing myself to others – women in particular – and my morale gets crushed. They all seem so much better off than me – physically, intellectually, and emotionally... All I feel fit for is a scrap heap.

Conflict and loss of control

Sufferers may have conflicting emotions such as the desire for control and the tendency to behave rashly; the ability to 'mother' other people, without being able to identify and meet their own needs first; a longing to be admired and wanted by a member of the opposite sex, and fears of making relationships:

> I'm tired of relationships that go nowhere. Most of the time I'm too tired and irritable to be bothered with giving or receiving attention, but deep down I think I really do want someone who can give me love and affection.

A great many sufferers are victims of a black or white way of thinking. They see themselves as either 'good' or 'bad' depending on the amount of willpower they have been able to exert over their eating. There are few grey areas in their outlook on life and their polarized way of thinking is reflected in the see-saw quality of their lives.

Apart from causing sudden mood swings, food cravings can prompt sufferers to behave rashly, particularly if they are surrounded by food when the urge to eat strikes. They may snatch it or, if they have no money, resort to shop lifting. Some experience a sort of hypnotic state when the desire for food is very strong, and in such cases there have been reports of sufferers grabbing food straight from shop shelves and eating it on the spot, much to the amazement of passers-by.

The depressing feeling sufferers sometimes get that their chaotic eating mirrors their inability to control their lives is not without reason. The impulsiveness with which they turn to food may affect other areas of their lives. They may rush out and buy clothes, cosmetics and jewellery in the same gratuitous way that they eat food.

> I'd get the urge to fill up the emptiness and sadness I felt inside. Usually I'd turn to food but sometimes I'd have a

spending spree on all sorts of baubles and trifling things–lipsticks, eye shadows, and trinkets. It all amounted to a small fortune which I didn't have, but I'd feel better for a while. I'd dash home in a flurry of excitement, try everything on, and end up feeling as lousy as ever. In between working overtime to pay off my overdraft, buying, bingeing, and vomiting, there wasn't much time for anything else, or even to really think about what I was doing.

Such sufferers can get deeply into debt. They then try to borrow from friends or relatives but cannot explain why they need the money. All this increases the feeling that their lives are out of control.

Depression and isolation

Some people think that bulimia is a depressive illness because sufferers sometimes seek help for depression before they need it for their eating problem. In many cases, however, it is difficult to establish whether the eating problem or the depression came first. The daily cycles of humiliating failure because sufferers have lost control over their eating can result in depression. Whatever the origins of their problem, the majority of sufferers end up feeling they are on a downward spiral.

Each day is a variation on the same theme of bingeing, vomiting and purging. All the time, effort and money I spend on my obsession is driving me to the brink of total disintegration.

Although bingeing and purging serve as a good excuse for avoiding life's pressures, many sufferers find that in time their sense of isolation increases. They become distressingly dependent on food as a panacea for everything and their method of coping with life turns out to be a very punishing regime. Horizons become increasingly narrow, and many describe feelings of being 'imprisoned', 'possessed', 'cornered', and 'trapped'. The world into which they have retreated eventually brings its own intolerable stresses of loneliness, lovelessness, fear, and depression. Many sufferers recognize that their eating habits are abnormal, and feel anger, loathing and aggression towards themselves. Some sufferers experience the kind of self-hatred that makes them despairing and suicidal. They may seek oblivion through an overdose of tablets. Some harm themselves by, for example, slashing their wrists. In such instances, admission to a safe environment such as a psychiatric hospital may be necessary.

When sufferers do seek help, they often find that much of their stress was caused by keeping their problem a secret. Ideally, professional help is given on an outpatient basis so that sufferers can retrain their eating habits and learn new ways of coping with their difficulties within their usual environment.

The pitfalls of hospitalization

Hospital medical staff whose professional role is to nurture and care for the sick tend to foster an atmosphere of dependence and compliance which can be damaging to bulimia sufferers in the long term. Those who are unable to face up to and deal with life's demands and challenges may come to rely on hospital staff for more than reassurance and support. They may shelve all personal responsibility and avoid facing up to their inner problems by adopting the role of a helpless victim who has been taken over by illness and needs to be cured. Bulimia sufferers must be prepared to accept responsibility for themselves and their behaviour, however, so a hospital environment may hinder their recovery.

Although many sufferers feel physically ill as a result of chemical imbalances (see chapter 7) and have a depressive outlook on life, the majority are not mentally ill in the same way that a victim of a psychotic mental disorder is. Manic depression and schizophrenia are examples of psychotic illnesses in which, during an acute phase, people lose hold of reality, have delusions and drift into worlds of their own making. Victims of these illnesses need hospital care and supervision until their symptoms are controlled. Although bulimia sufferers often find it difficult to concentrate and sometimes think in a disordered and distorted way as a result of their behaviour and preoccupation with food and weight, the majority remain lucid and fully aware of what is going on around them. The exceptions are when sufferers lose themselves in bingeing and talk about getting stoned or high on food, or they develop a severe secondary depression.

To sum up, therefore, bulimia sufferers are better off

receiving outpatient hospital treatment unless they are very run down, deeply and suicidally depressed and/or have an underlying psychotic illness.

An additional problem associated with going into hopital is the abruptness with which sufferers may be expected to give up their behaviour. Opportunities for bingeing are of course very limited in hospital, and sufferers for whom bulimia has become a way of life may find that having a sudden stop to their behaviour enforced upon them is like having the ground swept from under their feet. The shock will vary with individuals, depending on how long they have had bulimia, and on the nature of any background problems. For example, an underlying depression may become so overwhelming once the distractions of food/bingeing/purging are no longer immediately available, that sufferers become severely suicidal once they have entered hospital. Of course, depression can still afflict sufferers who are not in hospital, and this along with other factors which may influence recovery, is discussed more fully in Chapter 13.

4.

RISK FACTORS

The risk factors which can lead to bulimia include:
1. A tendency towards depression.
2. A tendency towards alcohol or drug dependency.
3. A biological predisposition to obesity.
4. Growing up in the western world with
   (i) its pressures to be slim;
   (ii) its conflicting messages about food;
   (iii) gender role conflicts.
5. A proneness to premenstrual carbohydrate craving.
6. Intolerance or hypersensitivity to certain food.
7. Certain physical illnesses.
8. Certain professions.
9. Abnormal brain chemistry.

Depression, alcohol, or drug dependency
It has been suggested that people with a tendency towards depression, alcohol or drug abuse may have a predisposition to developing bulimia. Studies have also shown that sufferers often come from families in which there is a high incidence of one or a mixture of these problems. No one knows exactly how or to what extent genetic and familial influences contribute to the development of the condition, but one theory is that sufferers learned to recognize the use of food, alcohol or drugs as diversions from stress when they were children.

Depression may be an underlying cause of bulimia, as has been explained, and sufferers themselves have drawn parallels with alcohol and drug dependency. Just as some essentially depressed individuals turn to drink or drugs as a mental painkiller, so others turn to binge-eating to give themselves relief from their emotional misery. Some sufferers turn to all three sources to produce temporary oblivion, and for those in whom depression may not have been a primary problem, it invariably arises as a secondary one because of the destructive cyclical nature of the disorder.

A biological predisposition to obesity

Some overweight individuals are not only more efficient at storing fat, even when they restrict their intake, but they also burn it up less effectively. It is thought they may run a risk of developing bulimia as a result of having to exercise a greater than normal control over their eating in order to become and stay slim.

Explanations for the difficulty such people encounter in losing weight relate to the 'fat cell theory'. Early feeding experience and hereditary factors influence the production of fat cells in the body. The number and size of these cells is thought to become fixed by about the end of the first year of life. Overfeeding in infancy, when new fat cells are being made, results in an excess production and a requirement for a high calorie intake in order to keep the cells 'topped up'.

Women to whom these background factors apply may not have been overweight as children because they needed plenty of energy while they were growing. After puberty, however, they needed less energy but continued to eat the same amount of food, so they put on weight rapidly. Satiety centres in the brain which control our appetite also tend to maintain the fat cell requirements at high levels throughout life, making it difficult for those to whom this applies to shift their weight problem.

Another consideration for overweight people who have to diet rigorously to lose weight involves the amount of brown body fat they have. People who lack this special type of fat, found mostly between the shoulder blades and around the kidneys, have a low metabolic rate and are prone to converting excess calories to fat, as opposed to burning them off. When they try to lose weight by dieting they often end up reducing their basal metabolic rate; that is, the speed at which the body uses energy to keep itself going in terms of warmth, growth and repair of body tissues, and functioning of vital body organs such as the brain, heart, liver, and kidneys. Once it has fallen, they have to restrict their food intake even further to continue losing weight. Thus many end up on regimes which are intolerably restrictive and impossible to maintain. Furthermore, people who deliberately keep their weight below that which nature intended it to be, and at which it functions best, often find that their yearnings for food become more intense and uncontrollable as their body continually strives to return to a naturally healthy 'pre-set' level.

Finally, studies have shown that the more that people on diets feel anxious about becoming fat, the more likely they are to indulge in sessions of over-eating as a result of the stress they are under. In time, this may put them at risk of developing bulimia.

Growing up in the western world

Pressures to be slim

> 'If you don't have first-class looks you stand a second-rate chance.'

This is a classic example of the sort of message which comes across in many glossy magazines and various other media outlets. A great deal of stress is put on women in western cultures because of the emphasis on the 'ideal' image or lifestyle which they are led to believe they ought to be training their sights on. The media messages are completely unrealistic, but they affect the opinions people have about themselves and others. Furthermore, they are primarily directed at women since they are the main consumers in society as well as the chief worriers about their appearance, size and weight. Fashion, diet and beauty industries brainwash women into thinking that there is only one approvable way of living, and those who do not conform to it are often made to feel inadequate. Advertisements brainwash the public into believing that fat equals unattractive, and youthful lissom 'women', who are in fact quite often adolescent girls, are used to advertise all the 'fun' things in life, from fast cars and exotic holidays to perfumes and boxes of chocolates. They are also portrayed in comfortable, salubrious surroundings, leading trouble-free lives, so it is not surprising that some women consider the only stumbling block between them and perfection is their physical appearance.

Women are urged, through avalanches of media advice, to develop 'firm', 'flab free', lithe and vibrant bodies. If they alter their physical characteristics, they are told, their lives will be transformed for the better. Apart from feeling happier with themselves, the insinuations are that they will be more commendable as people and more satisfied with life. Such propaganda undermines people's self-confidence. Adolescent girls who are going through a phase of increased sensitivity about their appearance and uncertainty about approaching adulthood, are especially vulnerable to such manipulative advertising. They may come to believe in it as 'the key' to personal, social and material success, and think that they can never be appreciated for their personality or intellect alone.

An additional source of strain for women in Western cultures is the extent to which the 'ideal' female shape has changed. This is well illustrated by comparing the appearance of celebrities such as film stars. During the 1940s and 1950s, women wanted a voluptuous, hour-glass figure like Jayne Mansfield and Marilyn Monroe. In the early 1970s, everyone wanted to be thin like Twiggy. Although this very thin figure is not so fashionable in the 1990s, with its emphasis on fitness and health, the ideal shape is still rather tubular, slim and flat-chested.

It is interesting to note that the so-called ideal form has always been the opposite of the shape that could be achieved easily. Thus for many centuries, women strove for a well-rounded figure and a well groomed appearance which emphasized their femininity – an ideal which was difficult to achieve when nutrition and hygiene were poor. Now, with abundant food supplies and aids to health care leading to a society of larger, taller, healthier, and more robust women the ideal is a slender boyish appearance and a denial of femininity. It is also interesting to note that this conflicting image is largely the product of female fashion – men have always preferred a well-rounded female figure.

In other societies such as India and the Middle East where this 'contrary' image has not been developed, bulimia and anorexia are far less common. However, when women from these societies become exposed to Western ideas and

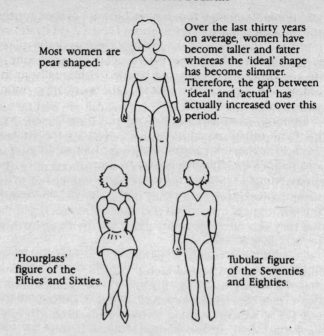

Most women are pear shaped:

Over the last thirty years on average, women have become taller and fatter whereas the 'ideal' shape has become slimmer. Therefore, the gap between 'ideal' and 'actual' has actually increased over this period.

'Hourglass' figure of the Fifties and Sixties.

Tubular figure of the Seventies and Eighties.

Figure 1: How Ideals Differ From Reality

culture, some do develop these disorders.

Men are now increasingly affected by the same pressure: to be slim is taken to correlate with being successful both socially and at work. If we look at the way men are portrayed in the media, it is clear that those who are represented as in some way successful nearly always have the 'lean and hungry look'.

Ignoring the media myth that life's problems will be solved by a trim figure is difficult even for the most clear-headed of people because this idea is often reinforced in the workplace, where thin people gain approval and promotion without too much difficulty: they tend to be seen as dynamic, strong-minded, and intelligent; and fat people tend to be discriminated against because they are associated with apathy, laziness and dullness.

Conflicting messages about food

Conflicting messages about food and eating put an

additional strain on women who, because of their nurturing role in society, have to think about food a great deal. On the one hand they are told they have a right to derive pleasure for themselves and to meet their needs through food, and on the other they are being warned continually to guard against food's potential for making them unhappy, unfit and unwanted.

Exciting, new, and miraculous diets, promising weight loss with minimum effort or discomfort are featured every week in various women's magazines, followed by pictures and recipes for delightful, easy to bake treats. As a result, many women worry continually about what they can and cannot eat, and it is not surprising that so many turn to dieting.

Gender role conflict

At one time, it was the acceptable norm for a woman to devote herself to creating a cosy home and rearing children, and she derived a sense of fulfilment from this nurturing role. Over the years, however, feminist movements have urged women to shake off 'the gentle sex' image and to learn to value their potential and abilities as independent, competitive, assertive, and liberated career women. Though they claim that they are trying to improve women's role in society, it has been suggested that the feminist lobby inadvertently places women in an ambiguous no win situation. Their ideology is poles apart from the conventional female attitudes and lifestyles, in which qualities of passivity, dependency, and compliance are predominant. Feminists argue that looking after a home and family is often mundane, demeaning and stultifying. Thus women find themselves in a dilemma. On the one hand they may feel committed to traditional feminine values, and on the other desire vocational success and achievement. The latter, however, entails joining the rat race, in which they may have to compete against men for promotion, carry a lot of responsibility, and be self-reliant and assertive. Furthermore, whilst such qualities are seen in general social terms to be valuable assets, in the context of the ideal woman – that is, someone who is decorative, compliant, not too intelligent and 'happy to take a back seat' – they are considered to be something of a liability and unfeminine.

Trying to reconcile these opposing traditional and feminist ideologies places great strain on women. Those who take on a job in addition to caring for the home and family not surprisingly feel physically and emotionally worn down at times. However efficiently they appear to juggle these two sets of expectations, there will probably always be a degree of inner turmoil and confusion about what they should do or be.

A proneness to premenstrual carbohydrate cravings

Hormonal changes during the premenstrual phase cause the amount of sugar in the blood to fall to abnormally low levels. Women who are particularly sensitive to these changes may experience cravings for sweet, high-calorie foods a few days before a period. In addition, the body's own protective mechanism for correcting the blood sugar levels may predispose individuals to binge-eating. Adrenalin is the hormone which is rapidly secreted to release sugar from the body's stores of glucose in order to restore the blood sugar to its normal levels. As it is also responsible for the 'fight and flight' reaction in humans, it may trigger off feelings of panic, tension and irritability. If this happens, eating may be a way of providing physiological as well as psychological relief by helping to temporarily blot out these distressing mental symptoms. Premenstrual physical discomfort in the form of headaches and a general feeling of bloatedness may also make some people seek solace by eating sweet carbohydrate rich foods.

Intolerance to certain foods

There has been increasing interest recently in the possibility that intolerance or hypersensitivity to certain foods, such as processed flour, wheat, chocolate and dried fruit, may constitute a risk factor for the development of bulimia. It is suggested that this causes a subtle and insidious allergic response, culminating in a vicious cycle of addiction. Larger and more frequent fixes are needed to get through the day and to prevent unpleasant withdrawal symptoms such as persistent tiredness, irritability, food cravings and panic attacks. Thus the bingeing syndrome might become established. This may be true for people who absorb these foods, but it is difficult to see how it could affect bulimia sufferers who make themselves sick and/or purge directly after eating.

Certain physical illnesses

Dr Hubert Lacey of St George's Hospital, London, has identified a group of patients with secondary bulimia[1]. These sufferers develop bulimia as a secondary disorder of a physical illness. He quotes diabetes and epilepsy as examples, and observes that the physical illness began at puberty – a time of heightened emotional tension – with the patient learning to be wary of certain foods which they know can trigger their symptoms. Subsequently, manipulation of food intake for emotional reasons develops.

Certain professions

Some professions place stringent demands on body weight, requiring a person to be as much as 10–15 per cent below the correct weight for their height and body frame. The obvious example is the slender model on the catwalk. Less obvious but equally pressurized groups include dancers, jockeys, airline cabin crew and athletes, who are often under a constant strain to keep within the limits placed upon them and may come to rely on vomiting after eating as a way of controlling their weight. In time this may lead to bulimia.

Brain biochemistry

Recent research has demonstrated abnormally low levels of a chemical called serotonin in bulimia sufferers. This substance is concerned with the transmission of nervous impulses between brain cells, and is particularly important in the area of the brain concerned with feelings of satiety (fullness after meals) and with the control of impulsive behaviour. Levels of this chemical have also been shown to be low in some individuals with depression. Antidepressant drugs which have been found to be useful in some bulimia sufferers are known to raise the levels of serotonin. It would seem therefore that in some cases, at least, a disturbance in brain biochemistry may be relevant to the development and maintenance of bulimia.

[1] 'Moderation of Bulimia', J. Hubert Lacey, *Journal of Psychosomatic Research*, Vol.28, 1984

5.

HOW IT STARTS

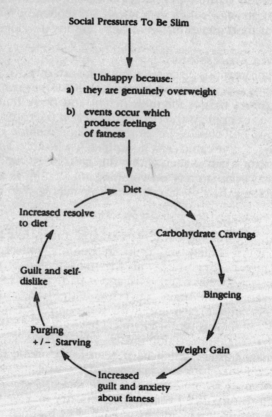

Social Pressures To Be Slim

Unhappy because:
a) they are genuinely overweight

b) events occur which
produce feelings
of fatness

Diet

Increased resolve
to diet

Carbohydrate Cravings

Guilt and self-
dislike

Bingeing

Purging
+ / − Starving

Weight Gain

Increased
guilt and anxiety
about fatness

Figure 2: The Binge/Purge Cycle

Binge-eating usually starts between the ages of fifteen and twenty-four. It may occur for one or more of the following reasons:

(i)   Social pressures to be slim (including a phase of anorexia nervosa)
(ii) An upsetting incident or personal remark
(iii) A major stressful event or adverse circumstance

Many sufferers have anxieties about fatness sparked off during their adolescent years by a personal remark concerning their shape, size or weight. They may be over-weight or simply think they are fat and develop a dislike for their body shape or size.

> I first became preoccupied with my figure when I heard my mother saying, 'She could be so attractive with those big brown eyes. It's a pity she's so plump.' I was fourteen then. When I next looked at myself I thought, 'She's right. I hate the size of my bottom and thighs.'

Social pressures to be slim spark off similar anxieties about fatness.

> I'd always been a chubby child and I got praised for having a clean plate. Mum encouraged us to 'eat up'. I'd eat whatever was put in front of me, whether I was hungry or not. By the time I was fifteen, food had come to play a major part in my life. I cycled daily to the sweet shop for supplies, weighed ten and a half stone and earned myself the nickname 'The Galloping Gourmet'. At about the same time I became interested in boys and pretty clothes. I wanted to have a silhouette figure, like the models, and hated being so plump and ungainly.

Pressure from people of their own age to look slim and attractive, and competing for the attention of someone of the opposite sex may also arouse fears about fatness.

> I unintentionally lost some weight one summer holiday and when I went back to school everyone complimented me on how much better I looked (I used to be known as Bessie Bunter). After that I felt I'd rather die than go back to how I was – being laughed at during games and so on.

> I had a crush on Peter and decided the only way to get him knocked out by me, instead of my friend Rosie, was to get stunningly slim. I went on a crash diet of black coffee and

cottage cheese (plus innumerable fainting fits) to jettison my
surplus flab as quickly as possible.

Breaking a semi-starvation diet of this kind is a common
triggering factor for initial binge-eating. Guilt, because the
body's need for more food overrides the desire to cut
down, may be considerable and items previously excluded
by the diet are often craved for.

> I'd eat nothing for four or five days and then gobble down
> everything I could lay my hands on. Food cravings seemed to
> threaten my sanity. I'd suddenly find myself wolfing down
> packets of biscuits, sweets, cakes, and sandwiches all in one
> sitting.

Initially binge-eating may have nothing to do with a
concern about appearance. In their late teens, girls may
begin eating for comfort because of stressful circumstances,
such as impending exams or an unhappy family
atmosphere, or because of conflicting feelings about leaving
the safety of home and becoming independent. Having to
rely on their own resources may prove to be more of a
strain than they had anticipated, particularly if they come
from an over-protective background.

> Moving away from home scared me stiff, even though I had
> been looking forward to it for ages. I wanted to prove to
> myself that I could cope with everything and the idea of
> having my own feelings, rights and responsibilities seemed
> great. Yet on my own I panicked. I felt out of my depth and I
> was inwardly terrified of having to fend for myself in a strange
> environment, not knowing a soul and feeling miserably
> homesick. I wanted to burst into tears and go running back to
> Mum. But I couldn't – not really – so I went to food instead.

An unhappy event such as a death or divorce, or illness
within the immediate family may also be a triggering factor.

> My grandfather died of a terminal illness. There had always
> been something special between us and having to watch him
> fade away was particularly upsetting. After he died I couldn't
> bear to talk about him to anyone. This feeling of loss grew
> inside me like a cancer. I went about like a bundle of gloom
> and would eat and eat and eat.

In older women, binge-eating may be provoked by a new
or unsatisfying job, a change of environment or the break-
up of an important relationship. The person may feel

deeply wounded and betrayed, and suffer a badly dented ego.

> Rob and I had been going out together for over a year. He was my knight in shining armour. I imagined he was going to fight all my battles for me and then whisk me away to some enchanted world of blue skies and sunshine. Then one day he went back to a former girlfriend and suddenly it was all over between us. I'd been magnetized by him, and without him my life was so empty. It seemed as if no one would ever take his place.

Women who have given up a career to look after the home and to have children may find that they miss the status and satisfaction of work outside domesticity. Feelings of isolation and the current low standing attached to being a housewife may generate a loss of self-esteem, feelings of resentment, loneliness, or boredom. The loss of financial independence is another consideration. Binge-eating may begin as a way of 'making up for all the self-sacrificing' they feel they do, or as a means of blanketing frustrations which make them feel guilty.

> I had this feeling of being nothing – of being crushed by domestic chores and the emotional demands of others. I was my husband's wife, my child's mother, my parents' daughter and I ceased to be a person in my own right. I felt resentful and increasingly fell back on bingeing to channel my mind away from this sense of imprisonment. It helped to fill the hollowness I felt about life, and the repetitiveness of it meant that I could drift from one grey day to the next with my brain in neutral.

Binge-eating may also begin as a source of solace for those who lack a warm and confiding relationship, particularly with a husband or boyfriend. They may constantly worry about what their partner thinks of them, feel restrained and uneasy about intimacy because they fear rejection, and put up with an unsatisfying relationship because they are unable to express their feelings, needs and desires.

Stressful events of the kind discussed, which involve a sense of loss, may provoke a reactive depression. For many sufferers, this is a major contributory factor to the development of their eating disorder.

6.

SIGNS AND SYMPTOMS

Irresistible urges to eat
The term bulimia, derived from the Greek 'boulimia–bous, ox + limos, hunger' and commonly described in the popular press as 'insatiable' or 'great' hunger, is a little misleading, since a characteristic feature of the condition is that sufferers over-eat irrespective of how hungry they are. Tension, loneliness, feelings of inadequacy, boredom, indecision and unexpressed anger are common precipitating factors, whereas hunger, despite dieting strictly in between bingeing, is seldom a predominant feature.

During a binge, sufferers experience a complete loss of control over eating:

> When I'm frantic for food my concentration slips. I get very frightened, irritable and upset. I liken myself to a robot that's been programmed to eat. Past experience tells me it's futile to fight the urge – my powers of reasoning vanish and I can't even think coherently.

Many feel a compulsion to eat large amounts of food, (carrier bags of it) over a relatively short period of time, such as two hours or less. Table 3 gives two examples of this. The food is often gulped down in a furtive manner and sufferers are ingenious at arranging circumstances or at finding safe places where they can binge and make themselves sick without discovery. The element of secrecy is also extended to the getting of the food so as not to arouse suspicion. Sweets and chocolates, for example, may be bought from several shops as opposed to bulk buying. Those who do buy food in large amounts from supermarkets may explain their purchases by pretending that they have a large family to feed or saying they are working in the catering business.

Table 3   Food Consumed During Typical Binges

1.	7.45–8.30 pm
	2 cheese sandwiches
	2 sausage rolls
	4 packets of crisps
	1 packet custard cream biscuits
	3 jam doughnuts
	2 Mars bars
	1 box Maltesers
	1 packet fruit pastilles
	1 litre lemonade
	$\frac{3}{4}$ box cornflakes, milk and sugar
	6899 Calories Vomited 6 times
2.	10.00–11.15 am
	1 loaf bread
	$\frac{3}{4}$ pot of jam
	$\frac{1}{4}$ pound of butter
	1 fruit malt loaf
	1 chocolate cake
	8 sausages
	1 pint of milk
	2 mugs of coffee
	$\frac{1}{2}$ pound vanilla fudge
	2 bowls of rice pudding
	8013 Calories Vomited 8 times

Expeditions for food may cause sufferers to become excited or anxious, and they sometimes abandon their shopping baskets or throw food away in a panic.

The initial stages of a binge are often enjoyable and sufferers feel relieved of tension. However, as more food is eaten, their sense of taste lessens or disappears altogether, and they experience a distressing loss of control.

I become dazed and unthinking. The control which I've had over my body seems to turn on me suddenly like a malevolent spirit, driving me on into my shameful ritual. Once I've embarked upon it I can't stop – it's as if I'm totally disconnected from myself and the world.

Many are overwhelmed by feelings of guilt, remorse and self-disgust:

I'm horrified at the sight of my painfully overstuffed stomach and feel like the nearest thing to a human pig.

High-calorie foods which are strictly avoided during phases of dieting are often selected to binge on, as are soft, easy to chew (and subsequently vomit) types of food. A few people begin bingeing on food which is highly coloured, such as oranges, carrots, or beetroot. They do this so that when they eventually make themselves sick they know when everything has been removed from the stomach.

Once they have lost control of their eating, sufferers will sometimes scour cupboard shelves and, in extreme cases, rubbish bins for edible scraps. They may also make up and eat bizarre concoctions of whatever ingredients come to hand.

I'd fly to the kitchen and make up unappetising mixtures of flour, water, oil, sugar, and eggs. When it was cooked it would turn into a thick rubbery mess, but I'd eat it just the same.

However, certain foods such as nuts may be avoided even during a binge because they are difficult to bring up.

Some binges are planned, leisurely affairs, for which food may have been hoarded. Other sufferers enjoy planning beforehand exactly which food they are going to buy for a binge:

I fantasize about all the food I'd most like to eat and then go off on a spending spree. At home I lay it all out in a particular manner, almost as if I'm going to entertain, and then plough my way through the whole lot.

For many sufferers, however, bingeing is laden with tension and anxiety because time and privacy may be at a premium.

During or towards the end of a binge, large amounts of fluid are often taken to mingle with the stomach contents and make the vomiting process easier. It also increases the abdominal distension and feeling of nausea, so that some sufferers feel they have a legitimate reason for making themselves sick.

Binge-eating may begin at any time of the day, though many sufferers find that they are more susceptible at certain times, such as at weekends or during the evenings. Episodes can last from fifteen minutes to a couple of hours and, depending on the available privacy, they may occur several times a day or just once or twice a month.

Sufferers who rely on fasting as a means of weight control tend to go through bingeing phases which may last for some days followed by several days of starvation 'to counteract the damage'. Those who practise self-induced vomiting and other forms of purging will often complete the binge/purge cycle within a couple of hours.

Bingeing usually stops when one or more of the following occurs:

(a)   Someone enters the room.
(b)   Food supplies run short.
(c)   Abdominal distension becomes intolerable, leading to vomiting.
(d)   The person feels too emotionally drained or physically weak to continue.

A lot of time and energy are lost on bingeing, but even more may be spent on thinking about how to avoid food, or about shopping or preparing for a binge.

Overwhelming fears of fatness

I dread the thought of how many calories all this food represents, but as I'm going to make myself sick, it doesn't really matter.

Sufferers are aware that unless they do something to counteract the nutritional effects of the food, they will gain weight. Faced with this worrying prospect they may adopt one or a mixture of the following methods of controlling their weight.

(i)   Fasting in between binges or dieting strictly.
(ii)   Taking 'handfuls' of laxatives to make food hurry through the intestinal tract in the belief that the

amount of calories absorbed and converted to fat will be minimized.
(iii) Taking slimming tablets (some of which contain laxatives).
(iv) Taking appetite-suppressant drugs such as amphetamines.
(v) Taking diuretic (water reducing) tablets to achieve a gratifyingly rapid weight loss. Only water is lost, but some sufferers believe that they 'melt' or flush fat away.
(vi) Excessive exercising.
(vii) Self-induced vomiting.

At first self-induced vomiting is often accomplished by pushing two fingers or some other object such as the handle of a toothbrush to the back of the throat. In time, some sufferers are able to regurgitate their entire stomach contents spontaneously by contracting the diaphragm and abdominal muscles. Making themselves sick may therefore become a fairly effortless and routine affair, which is not as offensive as vomiting because of a genuine stomach upset since binges are often returned in a relatively undigested state. Sessions may take up an inordinate amount of time, however, depending not only on the ease with which individuals can make themselves sick but also on the quantity of food to be disposed of, how meticulous they are about covering their tracks and their vomiting technique. Some sufferers adopt a rinsing out procedure to remove any residual stomach contents. This involves swallowing and regurgitating large volumes of water until it returns crystal clear. A very small minority resort to the dangerous procedure of inserting a tube down the oesophagus into the stomach as a means of giving themselves a stomach washout, demonstrating the degree of desperation they feel at the prospect of gaining weight.

Initially, vomiting and purging may seem like the ideal solution to the dilemma of how to combine eating with keeping slim. However, the practice is very habit-forming and after a while sufferers may consider a normal meal or minor over-indulgence sufficiently threatening to warrant a 'clear out'. Eating and vomiting may then become inseparable acts. Also, whilst self-induced vomiting starts in response to over-eating, it soon serves as a green light to abandon all dietary control.

When relief at having disposed of the food wears off, feelings of shame, humiliation and depression set in.

> After every session of bingeing and vomiting I see myself as totally reprehensible and unlikeable. If anyone shows me any kindness I regard it as a waste of their time and effort, and think that the world would be better off without me.

Most sufferers know that their eating is abnormal and promise themselves that they are never going to binge again. They make fresh resolutions about dieting and fitness but are haunted by fears that the compulsion to binge will return to overwhelm them, and that they will not be able to stop themselves. Their fears are not groundless. For some, the depresssion and self-dislike are so intense that the desire to binge is reactivated within a few hours.

7.

THE PHYSICAL AND EMOTIONAL SIDE-EFFECTS

The severity of symptoms will vary, depending on:
- (i) How long a sufferer has been practising bulimia.
- (ii) The body's capacity to tolerate and counterbalance the chemical disturbance.
- (iii) The frequency and regularity of the binge/purge behaviour.
- (iv) The quality of nutrition that is absorbed in between bingeing and purging.

Side effects of bingeing
The side effects of bingeing include:
- (i) Abdominal distension and pain.
- (ii) Swelling of the hands, legs and feet.
- (iii) Swelling of the salivary glands around the face and jawline.
- (iv) Tiredness, nausea, breathlessness, dizziness.
- (v) A pre-disposition to dental decay and gum disease as a result of bingeing on sugary foods.

Side effects of vomiting
These include the following disorders.

Hypoglycaemia (low blood sugar)
The normal response of the body to any carbohydrate intake is the secretion into the blood stream of the hormone insulin. The practice of self-induced vomiting results in an abrupt withdrawal of the carbohydrates which the insulin has been secreted to deal with, and it consequently has nothing to 'burn up' except the sugar which is present in

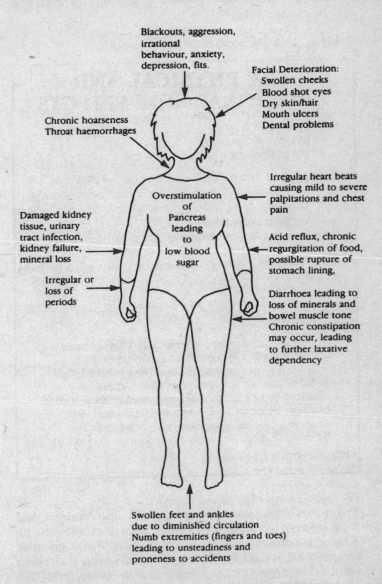

Blackouts, aggression, irrational behaviour, anxiety, depression, fits.

Facial Deterioration:
Swollen cheeks
Blood shot eyes
Dry skin/hair
Mouth ulcers
Dental problems

Chronic hoarseness
Throat haemorrhages

Overstimulation
of
Pancreas
leading
to
low blood
sugar

Irregular heart beats causing mild to severe palpitations and chest pain

Damaged kidney tissue, urinary tract infection, kidney failure, mineral loss

Acid reflux, chronic regurgitation of food, possible rupture of stomach lining,

Irregular or loss of periods

Diarrhoea leading to loss of minerals and bowel muscle tone
Chronic constipation may occur, leading to further laxative dependency

Swollen feet and ankles due to diminished circulation
Numb extremities (fingers and toes) leading to unsteadiness and proneness to accidents

Figure 3: Organs and Areas of the Body Affected by Bulimia

the blood stream. This causes the blood sugar to fall to abnormally low levels, producing a range of disabling symptoms (see Table 4).

Table 4 Hypoglycaemia (Low Blood Sugar)

Causes (related to bulimia)

1) Self induced vomiting
2) Prolonged fasting
3) Excessive exercising
4) Binge drinking of alcohol

Effects:

1) Sweating
2) Irregular heart beats
3) Epileptic fits / convulsions

4) Weakness / lethargy
5) Mental confusion
6) Irrational behaviour
7) Anxiety / panic attacks   Conducive to
8) Feelings of hunger   depression

The brain cannot store glycogen, (a form of sugar) and so its cells are dependent on an immediate supply of glucose in the blood. They need enough sugar to 'absorb' oxygen normally, and are very sensitive to lack of it. When this occurs, they cannot function properly and "nervous symptoms" arise. If there is a chronic sugar shortage, brain cells start to deteriorate, and long term brain damage may occur.

Chemical imbalance

Two important minerals, potassium and sodium are progressively lost from the body as a result of self-induced vomiting, laxative abuse or diuretic abuse. These minerals are essential for adequate muscle functioning and when their delicate balance is disrupted, debilitating metabolic complications can arise, see Table 5.

Table 5   Loss of Salt and Potassium from the Blood and Body Cells

---

Causes (related to bulimia)

1) Loss from gastrointestinal tract by:
   (a) self induced vomiting;
   (b) laxative abuse,
2) Loss through kidneys as a result of diuretic abuse

Effects:

1) Muscular weakness/lethargy
2) Tingling/numbness in fingers and toes
3) Confusion and poor concentration
4) Dehydration
5) Irregular heart beats
6) Low blood pressure
7) Kidney damage and further mineral losses

Dental problems
Stomach acid washing over the teeth wears away the enamel layer. The pulp and nerve endings may eventually be exposed and the teeth then have to be crowned. Dentists are often the first to question sufferers on their eating habits. Unfortunately, much of the salvage work undertaken to preserve a sufferers' teeth will be undone unless she stops using self-induced vomiting as a method of weight control.

Bleeding from the upper intestinal tract
Forced vomiting may be traumatic enough to cause blistering, tearing, and bleeding of the throat and oesophagus. In cases of severe trauma, rupture of the oesophagus has been reported, necessitiating major repair surgery (see figure 4).

Lack of protein
Self-induced vomiting and laxative abuse can result in a

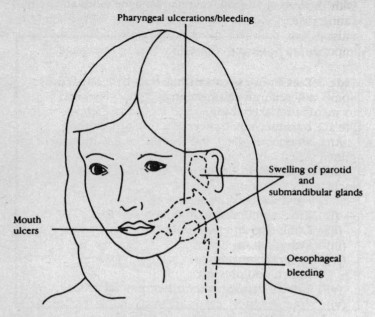

Figure 4: Effects of Bulimia on the Upper Intestinal Tract

shortage of protein. This causes an accumulation of water in the body tissues (oedema). Signs of oedema include a puffy face and ankles.

Side effects of laxative abuse

Sufferers who abuse laxatives soon feel extremely washed out and lifeless as a result of chemical imbalances which can threaten life if they are very severe. Chronic diarrhoea causes dehydration and a loss of body salts and minerals which may result in loss of muscle strength and heart irritability. Also, large intakes of laxatives may cause loss of bowel tone and secondary constipation which can propel sufferers into even greater laxative abuse.

When vomiting and laxative abuse are discontinued, sufferers may experience an uncomfortable sensation of fullness and bloating. Their stomach and ankles may also swell. These symptoms are usually temporary and are to do with the process of rehydration. When a normal diet and eating pattern is established, and the tone of the intestinal muscles has returned, the symptoms should subside. It is important to work out a withdrawal plan (see page 134).

Side effects of drug stimulants and alcohol abuse

Some sufferers use amphetamines ('pep pills') and alcohol to manipulate their weight and to divert themselves from life's pressures.

Amphetamines affect the central nervous system and mimic the effects of one of the body's hormones, adrenalin, which keys the body up for action. The initial effects include the following.

(i) Increase in energy.
(ii) Reduction in appetite.
(iii) A brightening of mood.
(iv) A reduction in the person's awareness of her surroundings.
(v) Lack of concentration.
(vi) Poor physical co-ordination and a proneness to accidents.

When the stimulant effect has worn off, the person feels irritable and confused, and a depressed 'hangover' occurs. This 'down' period may drive her to take another dose to return to the feeling of euphoria. Long-term effects include physical dependency, whereby larger and more frequent doses are needed to produce the desired 'high', hallucinations and feelings of being persecuted. In addition, as amphetamines are only available on the black market, they tend to be very expensive, and sufferers who are also supporting the habit of binge-eating may get hopelessly into debt.

Alcohol abuse produces a temporary feeling of triumphant well-being but, as with amphetamines, once the stimulant effect has worn off, depression sets in. Eventually, greater and more frequent amounts are needed to screen out reality.

Additional detrimental effects are listed over the page:

Table 6 Harm due to Intoxication

Medical problems	
Acute alcohol poisoning or overdose	Pancreatitis
Amnesic episodes	Trauma
Drug overdose	Head injury
Suicidal behaviour	Accidents
Acute gastritis	Epilepsy
Diabetic symptoms	Hangover
	Fetal alcohol syndrome
Social problems	
Social isolation	
Aggressive behaviour	Sexual problems
Passive behaviour	Domestic accidents
Domestic violence	Industrial accidents
Child abuse	Absenteeism
Child neglect	Poor time-keeping
Legal problems	
Driving offences	
Drunkenness offences	Criminal damage to property
Theft	Fraud
Shop-lifting	Deception
Taking and driving a vehicle	Assault
	Homicide

taken from *Drinking and Problem Drinking,* Dr. M.A. Plant, Fourth Estate Publishers, 1982.

The emotional aftermath

Depression as a cause and consequence of bulimia has already been discussed, and it is compounded by the fact that sufferers frequently have to lie, cheat, hide, or even steal in order to satisfy their urges to binge. Depending on the severity of the disorder, they may be prone to insufferable mood swings, particularly when urges to eat are very strong. They may become aggressive and intolerant of other people who they regard as being in the way, and such feelings often add to their sense of guilt. They also place great strain on relationships, thereby increasing their sense of loneliness and despair.

An additional source of friction which may contribute to the breakdown of relationships is the reckless way in which some sufferers spend money in an attempt to alleviate their unhappiness. Apart from running up enormous food bills, money may be frittered away on cosmetics and clothing.

About half the bulimia sufferers will have irregular or missed periods. Disruption of the menstrual cycle is thought to result largely from the stress and tension under which they are continually living, though chemical imbalances and large swings in body weight probably contribute.

Amenorrhoea and osteoporosis

Significant weight loss causes a decrease in the level of the female sex hormone oestrogen and an eventual loss of periods (amenorrhoea). Women in whom these changes have occurred become liable to a weakening of the bones and consequently an increased risk of fractures. This condition, known as osteoporosis, is commonly associated with post-menopausal women and the elderly but is now recognized to occur in younger women with a history of amenorrhoea and low calcium intake as a result of strict dieting.

Regaining normal body weight is usually accompanied in young women by a return of the menstrual cycle, but there is some evidence that there may not be a corresponding improvement in bone strength and density. Prolonged treatment in the form of oestrogen therapy and calcium supplements may therefore be advised in order to protect bones from weakening further and to prevent more bone loss. It is not yet clear whether this will result in bone density returning to normal, however, as these changes appear to depend upon the length of time a person has been severely underweight and amenorrhoeic. Osteoporosis is therefore more likely to be relevant to bulimia sufferers with a history of anorexia and amenorrhoea, although it is important to note that it does not necessarily occur in all those with such a background. Factors that appear to influence the likelihood of osteoporosis developing include the original strength of the sufferer's bones, exercise and an adequate intake of calcium. If you are concerned, discuss your worries with your doctor. A bone scan can be offered to assess the strength of your bones and to see whether treatment is indicated.

8.

KEEPING THE CYCLE GOING

Bulimia has some positive sides as well as many negative and unpleasant ones. It is worth acknowledging these in order to explain why, whilst desperate to put an end to their nightmarish existence, sufferers are often quite ambivalent about giving it up altogether.

The physical rewards of bingeing
Sufferers who binge on refined carbohydrates often experience 'highs' resulting from the instant boost of sugar to the brain via the blood stream. These highs lift their mood and make them feel all set for energetic activity, such as jogging, swimming or cycling.

The physical rewards of vomiting
Sufferers feel tremendous relief from physical discomfort, particularly from a distended stomach.

The emotional rewards of bingeing
More subtle ways in which the binge/purge cycle is perpetuated are to do with feelings and emotions. Whilst sufferers are so preoccupied with weight and food issues, there is little room for worrying thoughts or fears to be expressed. These are effectively blotted out by the bingeing process.

> I think about food nearly all the time. It's frightening to be so obsessed with it, but at least it stops me worrying about anything else.

Sufferers may turn to food so automatically that after a while they believe they have few other problems in life except those concerning eating and weight control. Once they look beyond their dietary problems, it can be very frightening for them to discover the stack of unresolved conflicts waiting to be dealt with and, not unreasonably, many think twice about taking the plunge towards recovery.

The problem with using food as a means of bypassing painful thoughts or uncomfortable feelings is that the less they are acknowledged and aired, the more fearfully alien they become, and the more the person depends on food and eating as a way of keeping them at bay.

Listed below are some examples which illustrate how bingeing can cocoon a person from the pressures and challenges of everyday living which they find it difficult to cope with.

Reasons for bingeing may include:

Pressure
I've had a day of pressures – it's my own way of relaxing and having 'time out'.

Anxiety
When I'm worried, eating helps to calm me down.

Concern about appearance
When I feel I'm fat, or getting fat, I get demoralized. I know I'll have to diet so I make up to myself whilst I'm allowed the food.

Confrontations
When I've had an argument with my boyfriend I think, 'Even if he doesn't love me I can still cosset myself with food'.

Boredom
When I'm bored it's a filler in of time, and a form of entertainment.

Self-punishment
The element of self-punishment may stem from the extremely low opinion sufferers often have about themselves. Many see themselves as totally unlikeable, and their lack of control about food confirms in their own minds that they are contemptible.

When my willpower snaps, I get even angrier with myself. Stuffing myself to the extent that I do is a way of getting at 'me', and all my faults, and I start thinking things like, 'Well, this serves you right, for being such a sap' and so on.

Bingeing may also serve as a way of eliciting attention and 'getting back' at people who sufferers think may have caused their problems in the first place. This also has the advantage of making them feel they are not responsible for their behaviour.

Other sufferers experience a pleasurable relief in the coming together of their mind and body when they binge. They no longer have to put up with internal conflict which arises when they are battling against the desire for food. However, this sense of physical and mental harmony only lasts as long as the initial stages of a binge. Once sufferers 'come to' and realize the extent of the damage, they are seized by panic and resort to desperate measures to try to turn the clock back.

The emotional rewards of vomiting and purging

Sufferers may feel some of the following emotions after purging.

(i)   A pleasurable sense of relief from physical distension and also from anxiety about absorbing too many calories.

(ii) A cleansing feeling:

It makes me feel physically and psychologically as if I've made an atonement for my sin of overeating.

(iii) A form of self punishment:

'Putting myself through this horrible performance is a way of getting back at myself for being so weak willed.'

(iv) A sense of security:

'I've always been horrified at the thought of becoming fat. Now when I want to eat I can do so without having to worry.'

Sufferers all have their own motivations for their behaviour. Being able to identify and find new and more productive ways of reacting to their emotions and needs is an important part of recovery.

Depression and premenstrual cravings have already been mentioned as a cause of bulimia and once the cycle has begun, they may help to keep it going. Dieting has been mentioned in the same context, as have chemical imbalances resulting from nutritional deficiencies and purging.

9.

SUMMARY OF WARNING SIGNS

1. Repeatedly avoiding meals. The person seldom wants to eat what others are having and says she will have something later on.
2. Visits to the bathroom shortly after a meal, ostensibly to have a bath or wash her hair.
3. Dramatic fluctuations in weight over a short period of time.
4. Mysterious disappearance of food.
5. Discoveries of sweet, cake or biscuit wrappers under chairs, pillows, mattresses or bedroom cupboards.
6. Continual overdrafts, debts and missing money. Inability to account for how it has been spent.
7. Frequent weighings. Talk about new diets and the wish to be thinner.
8. General dissatisfaction with appearance and figure. Expressing the wish to change.
9. Impromptu walks – often to buy food.
10. Night bird behaviour (so that she can binge when everyone else has gone to bed).
11. Increasing isolation, disinterest in social activities, work, studying.
12. General apathy and/or a depressive outlook on life.

10.

FAMILY INTERACTION

It is difficult for anyone living with a sufferer from bulimia to know how to confront the person about her behaviour. A warm, sympathetic approach in which you tell her what you suspect is probably best, but be prepared for flat denials and looks of wounded innocence. It may come as a shock to the sufferer to realize that she has been 'found out'. If she has been unable to face up to the problem herself, she will be reluctant to admit it to anyone else. Fear of rejection will always be uppermost in her mind. This is why, however infuriated you may feel about her denials, it is best to avoid being authoritarian, coercive or condemnatory in an effort to get her to seek help. You will probably feel justifiably angry about being cheated, lied to or used, and about the waste issue, but giving full vent to these feelings will, in the long term, be counterproductive. The sufferers's eating habits are likely to become more secretive, and she may develop an even greater tendency to seek solace in food. Alternatively, she may agree to see a doctor to appease you, but feel full of resentment, contrariness and reluctance to co-operate, none of which will pave the way for a lasting recovery.

This does not mean that you have to concede that there is nothing wrong, however. You can remind the sufferer frequently that you know what is going on, that you are involved in her misery, and that you are ready to lend support and encouragement when she finally decides to seek help. You can explain how distressing it is to watch a person ruining her life and making other people's lives a misery too.

All this may appear to fall on deaf ears, but those who are

prepared to confront their problem will probably take what is said to heart. Waiting for them to acknowledge that they need help can be a frustrating time, but in the long run it is vital that they decide this for themselves and that they feel personally motivated to work towards a recovery.

Apart from the issue of confronting sufferers with their behaviour, family and friends of bulimia victims are often desperate to 'help' a sufferer to recover. They may go to such extremes as removing bathroom doors, patrolling the kitchen, keeping inventories of food or padlocking the fridge in the misguided hope that their efforts may make it easier for the sufferer to control herself. This sort of intervention, well-intentioned as it may be, can lead to an escalation of despair as sufferers tend to react by becoming more difficult or more dependent. Feelings of anger, humiliation or frustration not uncommonly manifest as more deranged eating patterns, leaving friends or relatives with the pain and guilt of having apparently made things worse. Other families find that in assuming the role of a caretaker or guardian, they have inadvertantly fostered a sense of helplessness whereby the sufferer relinquishes all responsibility and looks to others to put things right. It is important to understand that there is little that can be done for a bulimia victim that will necessarily make her better. The process of change must come from within. Encouragement and support are vital but the sufferer must be given the chance to realize that she can act effectively on her own behalf.

PART II

A PLAN FOR RECOVERY

In their attempts to recover from bulimia, some sufferers will decide to 'go it alone'; others will reach out for professional help and support. Whichever avenue they choose, it is hoped that the second part of this book will convey a message of hope and optimism, and instil sufferers with confidence in their own ability to help themselves. Various strategies are offered to help them overcome their difficulties about food and to inspire them to try better ways of coping with life's stresses. What one sufferer finds beneficial may be of less value to another, and as each individual's circumstances are unique, the intention is that readers select and perhaps modify those ideas which they think will best suit them.

11.

LAYING FOUNDATIONS

Acknowledging difficulties

An important though often painful first step is for you to admit to yourself that your eating habits and behaviour about food are not normal. This will strike some sufferers as obvious, but others have been caught in the bulimia cycle for several years, and their behaviour has become second nature. These people may have become blind to its consequences for themselves and for other people.

What often makes this step such a difficult one to take are the guilt and shame felt about a habit which is socially unacceptable. Many sufferers regard their own behaviour as disgusting and are so afraid of rejection by other people that it may be years before they are finally able to face up to their difficulties and seek help. They may decide to sit tight, hoping that if they try to discount their behaviour it will resolve itself in time. Some stumble painfully from one year to the next in the belief that when they eventually decide to stop they will be able to do so at a stroke.

Little is known about the natural course of bulimia, because it is such a secretive condition. But, as with any problem allowed to develop over a lengthy period, it will inevitably take some time to overcome. This is why it is important for you to acknowledge your difficulties as early as possible, and to obtain help if this is what you want. If you are using food as a mechanism for coping with strain, you may not wish to tackle the greater strain of trying to do without your prop. However, denial of the problem does nothing to solve it. The longer you remain trapped in this chain of problem eating, the harder it becomes to break free, and the more frightening the prospect of change.

Taking personal responsibility

It is also essential to guard against the unhelpful notion that someone should, or could, resolve your difficulties for you. This means having the courage not only to face up to the problem, but also to take responsibility for yourself and your condition. You must refuse to allow yourself to become a victim of the past and pin all the blame for your unhappiness on parental weaknesses, poor upbringing, unfortunate episodes and so on. If you say, 'I have been moulded by my past and therefore cannot be anything other than I am,' you are really saying 'I am not to blame for my behaviour and I am powerless to change it'. This makes you feel helpless and unable to control your own destiny, and despair and despondency meet you at every turn. Whatever happened to you in years gone by, it is important to believe that if you really want to, you can call a truce with the past and move towards a better quality of life.

This does not mean, however, that by turning to someone else for help you are trying to evade all personal responsibility. Rather, it is an indication that you have realized the extent of your difficulties, and that you feel determined to deal with them.

Keeping an open mind

Seeking a lasting recovery from bulimia often calls for a great deal of perseverance, open-mindedness, flexibility, and courage. You must be willing to try out different ways of overcoming the triggering factor which causes you to binge, whether it is boredom, anxiety, anger, frustration, or a mixture of such miseries. If one approach fails be prepared to move on to another until you find one which is right and really works.

Keeping to the truth

Honesty is the best policy. Presenting a distorted picture by colouring the truth or by glossing over it with veiled hints such as 'sometimes I eat too much', or 'I sometimes feel sick', may result in being offered inappropriate help. Being truthful should help you to establish a good relationship with the person you are confiding in. This is crucial because if you ever do reach a stage of feeling desperate about things, you will at least have someone to whom you can unburden yourself freely and without concealment.

12.

REACHING OUT

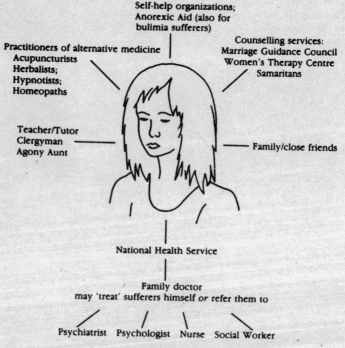

Figure 5: Reaching Out for Help

Various agencies, self-help organizations and professionals who may be able to offer support of differing kinds are listed below. Most of them encourage individuals to look afresh at their outlook on life. By listening, and trying to share their feelings without passing judgement, these agencies and professionals can help sufferers to make their own decisions rather than pressing advice or making decisions for them. Although obtaining the understanding and supportive help of relatives and friends is valuable, particularly if you have dreaded rejection, they are not always able to give unbiased and dispassionate opinions. It is therefore very useful to confide in someone who is not involved in your personal life. An outsider will be better able to see your problems in a neutral light and to make suggestions about tackling them.

The family doctor

The family doctor is usually one of the first people sufferers think of approaching for help. When making an appointment there are a few useful points to remember.

1. Ask the receptionist for a double appointment, preferably at a time when the surgery is not too busy. Bulimia is not a condition that can be explained properly in a few minutes and if the doctor has a lot of patients waiting, you may not receive his full attention.
2. Make a note in advance of all the things you want to tell and ask the doctor, including any worrying physical symptoms. It is easy to forget things when you are nervous and upset.
3. Don't be afraid to jot down what the doctor says, such as what is on offer in the way of help, and any alternative options and tests which are suggested. The doctor should not mind, and again, if you are tense and worried, you may not remember what you are told.

What to expect from the doctor

Responses from family doctors vary with the training they have had in counselling work. Some seem to be fairly intolerant of people suffering from complaints of an emotional origin, particularly if they regard these as self-inflicted, whilst others take the time to listen to patients who need to unburden themselves. If your family doctor is the type who reaches for the prescription pad before you have even finished talking, or adopts a 'pull your socks up' attitude, it is worth asking to be referred to someone else, or taking the initiative of changing to another practice. Suggestions for how to go about this are given below.

Try not to let an abrupt or dismissive manner put you off seeking other help. You can ask to be 'released' from the practice. You do not have to explain why. You can find out about other general practitioners in the area by:

(a) looking in the Yellow Pages under the heading 'Physicians and Surgeons';

(b) asking the administration office of your local health board or family practitioners committee to advise you about doctors in your area. Look for the headquarter's telephone number in the telephone directory under the heading 'Health'; for example, 'The Lothian Health Board – Area Board Headquarters';

(c) asking friends or neighbours if they know of a doctor who is considerate and prepared to listen – most receptive doctors acquire a good reputation.

Changing practices can involve having to take several leaps of faith before you find someone you are happy with. Despite this, it is worth making the effort. Getting the right help and understanding can mean the difference between sinking or swimming.

Formalities for changing doctors

Procedures have been simplified and it is now no longer necessary to obtain written permission from your practitioner or to wait for registration. Remember also that under no circumstances do you have to give your reason for wanting to change.

A family doctor who is sympathetic but unfamiliar with the condition of bulimia may decide to refer you to the outpatient clinic of a specialist in eating disorders. If there is not a specialist in eating disorders in your area, the doctor may refer you to a general psychiatrist. Eating disorders have become a regular part of psychiatric care, so if this is suggested try not to feel ashamed or alarmed by it. The prospect of going along to a psychiatric hospital may be daunting, but it is usually worth attending for at least one appointment. An informal discussion with a psychiatrist or with one of his back-up team (which might include a psychologist, a nurse and/or a social worker) is generally used as the first line of help. You can then go away with a clearer idea of the available options.

Hospital help

As discussed earlier, unless you are severely physically run down, have some other psychiatric problem, or are very depressed, you will probably be treated on an outpatient basis. This is so that your chaotic eating pattern, which may have been caused by a mixture of social and personal problems can be looked at and tackled constructively within your everyday setting.

Broad aims of the treatment will generally include helping you to:

   (i)   develop normal, more relaxed attitudes to food and weight;
   (ii) stop using abnormal and potentially dangerous methods of losing weight;
   (iii) stabilize your weight at a 'natural' level;
   (iv) identify certain moods such as boredom and anxiety which propel you to binge-eating;
   (v)   identify specific aspects of your life which precipitate bingeing, such as an inability to enjoy spare time in a relaxed or personally fulfilling way, lack of close friends, insufficient interests aside from your work, depression and so forth;
   (vi) devise more productive ways, other than over-eating, of reacting to life's stresses.

What might you be offered?

Broadly, you may be offered any of the following courses of treatment.

   (i)   Psychotherapy or 'talking treatment'.
   (ii) Group therapy.
   (iii) Behaviour therapy.

(i) **Psychotherapy.** The essence of this is that you build up a personal relationship with the therapist by talking, usually for an hour once a week. However, hospitals vary in what they offer, and therapy with a busy psychiatrist can, unfortunately, turn out to mean half-hourly sessions once a fortnight or month. This can seem like an eternity if you are feeling very low, so it is worth asking if there is someone you can get in touch with between appointments should you start to feel bereft of hope. Over a number of weeks the therapist will guide you to talk as freely as you can about a variety of issues. The sort of topics normally include:

(a) your childhood experiences;
(b) the work you do now;
(c) how you get on with other people;
(d) where you live;
(e) sexual relationships;
(f) your feelings;
(g) the underlying motives for your behaviour, including your eating pattern.

A large proportion of psychotherapy will consist of the therapist simply listening to what you say. Whilst doing this she will try to enter into your world of feelings so that she can understand exactly what it is like to be in your shoes. At the same time, it is important that she retains some objectivity about your situation so that she can help you to understand the nature and cause of your problem. Many emotional and physical symptoms arise from a denial of feelings. Therapists therefore aim to help you to uncover, express and accept your true emotions instead of guiltily storing them away and pretending that you feel something else. Thus, you can come to see yourself, other people and the world in a new light. In addition, therapists aim to provide a supportive and accepting role, regardless of what you say or tell them. This is essential for winning your trust and enabling you to talk openly about your experiences, behaviour and feelings. It is important, however, to note that being supportive does not entail sending you away with a list of do's and don'ts. Rather it is a process of encouraging you to believe in yourself as a worthwhile person and to explore and discover your own strengths and weaknesses. All this adds up to developing a clearer understanding and awareness of yourself. Having achieved this, you are then encouraged to accept personal responsibility and to experience the satisfaction of finding your own means of combating your problem, as opposed to having answers prescribed.

People undergoing psychotherapy often worry about the question of confidentiality. Therapists normally make an effort to assure them at the outset that whatever they say will be treated in the strictest confidence. However, there may be occasions when a therapist feels it would be in a patient's interest to discuss the case with a colleague, and in such instances the person is almost always told beforehand. It is worth noting that psychotherapy in the National Health Service is different from psychoanalysis which is usually only available privately. Analysis may take years and cost a great deal of money. It is expensive and several weekly sessions are usually required so that the analyst can find out all he can about a patient's personality. Psychotherapy through the NHS is not nearly as drawn out or deep reaching, but this does not mean that it is any less valuable for people who need to talk to someone about their innermost fears and turmoils.

(ii) **Group therapy.** Psychotherapy can be conducted effectively in a group. The benefits include a sense of belonging and the realization that there are others in the same boat with whom you can share your feelings. Practical ideas can be exchanged and, as a result of lending support to each other, members can come to realize that they still have some value in spite of their difficulties. These factors can contribute a great deal to improving a person's sense of self-worth and restoring a shattered self-confidence, as well as easing feelings of isolation.

(iii) **Behaviour therapy.** Many psychiatrists do not categorize bulimia as a mental illness. They regard it as a learned behaviour which has become a habit. The idea behind behaviour therapy is that you can unlearn an unwanted pattern of behaviour with appropriate guidance. The focus is not so much on what makes you tick, as on your external behaviour.

The therapist will try to help you to pinpoint triggers to binge-eating, such as boredom, bottled-up anger, loneliness; give practical assignments to help you to regain control of your eating and encourage you to find more productive and fulfilling ways of coping with life.

Although behaviour therapy does not concentrate on underlying emotional problems to the same extent that psychotherapy does, it can be valuable for bulimia sufferers who have developed a conditioned response (bingeing) to stressful situations and emotions. During therapy, triggering factors for your behaviour will become apparent, and having identified these, it is possible to re-train your reactions to them.

All these forms of therapy can help you to get to grips with your eating, and are worth trying if they are offered. You have nothing to lose, and having someone to talk openly to about your bulimia will help to remove much of the fear and guilt associated with harbouring a dark secret.

Remember, however, that therapy in any form is not infallible and it would be wrong to expect it or your therapist to cure you. People who put responsibility for their recovery onto someone else are often bitterly disappointed. Furthermore, the best treatment in the world is not going to make much of an impact on you if you lack the determination and resolve to face up to and overcome your condition.

On the other hand, therapy will probably help to set the course for recovery and follow-up appointments offered by most therapists at the end of treatment can serve as powerful incentives for you to consolidate what you have learned.

The issue of honesty as an important prerequisite for recovery has been stressed and it is important not to feel that you have to present yourself to your therapist as a cured case as your treatment nears completion. If you do not feel that you are better, you should say so. This may seem obvious, but bulimia sufferers tend to want to please others and this may make them exaggerate their progress. Therapists can normally assess an individual's true progress for themselves, of course. Many of them know that patients sometimes feel under pressure to win their approval and they make allowances for this in their progress assessments. Even so, they cannot guess at everything if the patient does not tell the truth.

Therapists are of course delighted when their patients make full and speedy recoveries, but most of them understand that individuals differ enormously in the time it takes them to overcome their difficulties. They will not think any the less of you if you have not made a complete recovery by the end of treatment. Successful treatment is often assessed on how well you can control and manage your symptoms, rather than by a complete cessation of them.

So try to stay above board at all times and keep your therapist fully in the picture with regard to your real progress. After the relief of admitting to someone that you have a problem, it can be very depressing to feel yourself backsliding into a tangle of deception purely as a result of wanting your therapist's approval.

Apart from keeping your conscience easy, being honest will ensure that if you are unfortunate enough to experience a severe setback later on, and want support, you will not lose face after having apparently done so well. Remember that you are getting better because you want to and not to please your therapist.

What about drugs?

As yet there is no medication to 'cure' bulimia in the same way that a person with, say, a chest infection will recover after a fortnight's course of antibiotics. Neither is there a drug that will prevent sufferers from placing too high a value on being thin or from holding on to the concept that their lives will be transformed for the better when they have attained an 'ideal' body shape which may border on emaciation.

Trials are in progress, however, to evaluate the role of anti-depressant drugs in managing the food cravings and depression that sufferers commonly experience. The majority of published studies have demonstrated that the use of anti-depressants is associated with a significant decrease in binge frequency, so it is likely that these drugs will feature more prominently in future regimes for bulimia sufferers. At present it is impossible to distinguish which sufferers will respond to anti-depressant therapy; also unknown is how many will relapse when the drugs are stopped. In general, however, anti-depressant drugs are thought to be of more benefit to sufferers who are prone to down swings of mood of a chemical origin or disturbed hormone balance (endogenous depression) than for the more common type of 'reactive' depression which occurs in response to life events, such as disappointments, repeated rejection or problems at school or work.

An important point to bear in mind when starting any anti-depressant medication is that an improvement in mood and outlook will not generally begin to occur until a therapeutic level of the drug in the blood has been attained. This often takes two to three weeks. Perseverence may therefore be necessary in the early stages of treatment when, in the absence of immediate results, sufferers may be tempted to stop taking their tablets.

People often have reservations about taking anti-depressant drugs in case they experience unpleasant side effects or become dependent. With controlled use, however, they can be helpful, particularly in the early stages of recovery when depression may result either as the emergence of an underlying trend or as a new event. Severe depression, if untreated, can make it difficult for you to feel motivated enough to tackle your bulimia, let alone any of the underlying causes of it. However, you must decide for yourself whether or not you want to take anti-depressant drugs. Use your common sense. If you decide against it make sure that your doctor understands your views on the subject.

One drug which seems to show particular promise for the treatment of bulimia is Fluoxetine (trade name: Prozac). This drug can be used in low doses to treat depression and in higher doses (60 milligrams a day) to treat bulimia. Studies have shown that when Fluoxetine is used in the treatment of normal-weight bulimia sufferers, approximately 25 per cent will stop bingeing and vomiting after taking the drug for eight weeks. The beneficial effects of the drug may not be sustained, however, unless it is used as part of a treatment plan that includes dietary counselling and psychotherapy.

The side effects of Fluoxetine vary but common complaints include nausea, lethargy, loss of sex drive and difficulty in sleeping. There has also been unsubstantiated speculation in the USA that it may give rise to violent or suicidal behaviour.

Sources of help outside the National Health Service

Help may be obtained from a variety of voluntary local

counselling services and self-help organizations, most of which emphasize personal responsibility. Counselling is a less intensive form of psychotherapy. Good counsellors will try to help you towards a more realistic outlook on life and the things you value without giving specific advice.

The following organizations may be able to help you. Addresses and telephone numbers are given on pages 145–146.

The Samaritans (the befrienders)
They also describe themselves as 'the listening ear'. You can talk to them personally or ring them up about a problem without giving your name. They do not provide any formal treatment, but if you are feeling depressed, a sympathetic ear can help to combat despair.

Relate (The Marriage Guidance Council)
Marriage guidance is a misleading name, since nearly all services will see individuals, particularly if they are one of a married pair. It aims to provide a service that will help people to deal with their lives and relationships more effectively.

The addresses and telephone numbers of local branches of the Samaritans and Relate can be obtained from the telephone directory or from your local Citizens Advice Bureau.

The Women's Therapy Centre
This organization is based in North London and is run by therapists with feminist views. They offer help for various eating disorders and are prepared to give advice to anyone interested in setting up a self-help group.

The Maisner Centre for Eating Disorders
This centre is run by Paulette Maisner, who for years suffered from compulsive eating. It aims to help people with compulsive eating problems and bulimia. A selection of courses are offered, all of which are based on the Maisner Method. This comprises a mixture 'of relaxation therapy, guidance on nutrition, and special dietary needs, and a sympathetic ear'. Talking to someone who, as they say, has 'been there' is undoubtedly of help to many sufferers, and

because of the success of her method, Paulette is hoping to set up new centres around the country. Brochures are available on request, detailing the precise nature and cost of each course.

Self-help organizations

Information about these organizations can be obtained from the organizations' headquarters; women's health shops; Citizens Advice Bureaux; libraries; or the Samaritans.

There are local as well as national self-help groups and sufferers can find out about relevant ones in their area from any of the above sources.

The Eating Disorder Association (EDA)

This charity is an amalgamation of Anorexic Aid and Anorexic Family Aid which formerly worked independently. The Association offers help with all forms of eating disorder, especially anorexia and bulimia. It is able to provide support through a national network of self-help groups, telephone help lines, written guidelines and newsletters. Research and exchange of information is also provided in a journal which is published bi-annually, entitled *Eating Disorders Review*.

Details are given in the Useful Addresses section at the back of the book.

All these groups try to explore and deal with pressures which cause, perpetuate and prolong bulimia, and also provide companionship, moral support and encouragement for sufferers. Many people are relieved to have somewhere that they can talk freely and know they are not alone:

It was reassuring to know I was not the only one, and a relief to talk to other women who understood the full horror of bulimia.

Members are often at different stages of recovery and those further on can give helpful leads to those just starting out.

Alternative medicine

Alternative medicine is becoming increasingly well known, and you may find this approach very helpful. You could consult a practitioner of herbalism, acupuncture or homoeopathy, for example, but perhaps the most appropriate would be a hypnotherapist.

Hypnosis entails being deeply relaxed by the therapist. Whilst in this state of 'altered consciousness' the patient is more open to therapeutic suggestions. There is no doubt that hypnosis can relieve people of anxieties and fears and mild addictions such as cigarette smoking, but it has its limitations. Successful treatment depends on a number of factors, including how suggestible you are, and the skill of the therapist. It is also generally believed that hypnosis cannot make a person do something that they do not really want to do, or which goes against their 'moral code'. This means that unless you really want to give up your behaviour, hypnosis will probably be of little value. Another consideration is that it involves a high degree of dependence. Consequently, you may rely on the therapist to 'cure' you and lose all motivation to help yourself.

Whichever of these forms of treatment you choose, it is important to ensure that you go to someone who is properly trained and experienced. Try to see someone who has been recommended to you, and always check on their credentials.

Most forms of treatment have a recognized organization which can help you to find a reliable practitioner. There are many books available where you can find the address of such organizations.

13.

SOME STUMBLING BLOCKS

Recovering from bulimia is hard work, well described by some sufferers as an 'uphill slog'. Some of the most testing hurdles are encountered fairly early on, and those who have recovered can remember having had to endure a certain amount of misery before getting better.

> I had come to rely on food and eating to the point where it took over my life. Trying to cut it out threw me into a state of sheer panic, which made me feel I was going from bad to worse.
>
> I didn't expect to knock up against so many difficulties as a result of giving up my behaviour. The depression was the worst. Each day seemed to be a grinding struggle in which I wanted to throw in the towel and accept that I was beaten. After about five weeks things began to take a turn for the better. The dark days became fewer and my progress began to quicken.

A major difficulty is the fact that you need food. You cannot turn your back on it in the same way that you could with alcohol or cigarettes. You need to eat in order to live, and since it is food which both provokes and aggravates your disorder, retraining your eating habits can be particularly stressful.

Another dilemma frequently encountered is the discovery that you are in two minds about giving up your behaviour. You may feel very frightened about what you are doing to yourself, and want to change, but at the same time you are terrified of the consequences of eating normally.

> I envisaged bulging at the seams and putting on pound after pound of excess baggage.

Blowing hot and cold about recovery can also create conflict for you if you derive something positive from your behaviour, such as a release from boredom, a form of entertainment, or a way of getting from day to day without feeling too emotionally knocked about. You may have come to feel comfortable within your preoccupying existence with food. Restrictive though this is, it promotes a sense of security. Susie Orbach, author of *Fat Is a Feminist Issue, 2* (Hamlyn, 1982), explains:

> A binge is predictable. You are familiar with the course it takes. It leads you through a pattern of emotional responses that you have come to know ... and it allows you to temporarily absent yourself from distress.

As a result of relying so much on food to get themselves from day to day, some long-standing sufferers lose all ability to solve their problems in a clear-headed way. Rather than have to look for new ways of tackling old challenges, they tend to take the view 'better the devil you know'. If this applies to you, one way of persuading yourself to change is to remember that few things in life are completely irreversible. Taking a step into the unknown, even for a limited period of three or four months, may turn out to be more profitable than doing nothing. If you do not like the outcome you can always return to your old ways.

A third common stumbling block is the worry that whoever you turn to for help will reject you. Many sufferers are aware of the difficult and lonely struggle which lies ahead of them, and want help from their family and friends, but are haunted by the question 'will they still like/love me if I tell them?'

There is no doubt that telling others about your difficulties will involve a painful self-exposure, but the only way to begin to solve a problem like bulimia is to admit it is happening in the first place. A reassuring thought is that people who have been closely involved in your life will probably be relieved to discover that there is a reason behind the baffling emotional storms they have had to put up with. Consequently, their reaction will be much less condemnatory than you feared. Also, it is worth trying to remember that it is the behaviour itself which relatives or friends disapprove of, rather than you as a person. Plucking up the courage to tell someone close is therefore a painful but crucial step to take, enabling you to obtain practical help and to relieve yourself of the anguish of carrying a guilty secret.

Depression can be another barrier, and it is not unusual for sufferers to find that they feel worse before they feel better.

> Giving up bulimia seemed at times to be a brutal struggle – I hadn't counted on being so depressed.

Although your eating may have begun to stabilize, it may suddenly dawn on you how much time, energy, suffering and money has been spent on bingeing, purging and/or starving. Furthermore, you may feel at a loss to know how to fill the void left by the removal of something which had become a way of life. If you have become so preoccupied with food and eating, to the extent that you feel you sometimes function 'as a robot', you may also feel distressingly vulnerable and emotionally naked or raw when you cut down the frequency of your bingeing. For the first time in months, or even years, you may suddenly find yourself aware of the capacity to feel. Anger, anxiety, jealousy, loneliness and sadness will be feelings which are frighteningly unfamiliar because they have been buried under incessant thoughts of dieting, weight, food and bingeing. However, it is only by becoming more emotionally aware that you will be able to confront and resolve unconscious conflicts.

Some sufferers are able to adapt to 'feeling human' again quite quickly, whereas others take a while to adjust. If you have long been entrenched in bulimia, guard against feeling a failure if it takes longer than you expected. A few sufferers claim to have given up bulimia straightaway, but many others are unable to make this sort of clean break from their pattern of behaviour. Trying to kick the habit abruptly is simply too upsetting, for the reasons outlined. Therefore, weaning yourself away from your behaviour, inch by inch, hour by hour, day by day, can help to sidestep the frightening feeling of being swamped by a downpour of emotions. At the same time, you can start to adapt to alternative ways of coping with life's stresses in a manner and at a pace which suits you.

14.

IT IS NEVER TOO
LATE TO CHANGE

There are probably many times when you feel exasperated and so demoralized by your own behaviour about food that you seriously wonder 'will I ever be able to eat like a normal person again?' The answer can by 'yes', providing you are prepared to work at it in the ways outlined below. Getting back to normal is for many sufferers a step-by-step procedure of retraining their minds and stomachs to accept a more conventional eating pattern. Perseverance is needed to take the setbacks that are part of any rehabilitation process. Bad days do not automatically cancel out any progress achieved. Being gentle on yourself and learning to acknowledge your successes is just as essential as being determined and patient.

On the food front
In order to get to grips with your eating it is a good idea to give up dieting, since it invariably causes and perpetuates difficulties with food. Women who have got over bulimia are often able to see how futile their efforts were to alter their body shape and weight by crash or 'fad' dieting.

> I became plagued by thoughts of food and eating to the exclusion of all else – I read about food, I talked about it, I entertained myself with it, I beat myself up with it and I even dreamt about it. It eventually created more problems for me than it solved. Hardly a day went by when I wasn't submerged by either dieting or gorging.

Despite its drawbacks, the mere suggestion of giving up

dieting can cause tremendous anxiety. You may be convinced that when you eat normally you will gain an immense amount of weight. One way of easing your apprehension is to think of the three or four months ahead of you as an experiment in which you plan to give up dieting. Studies have shown that everyone has a naturally healthy 'set point' weight. This weight may fluctuate by four or five pounds a month depending on factors such as pre-menstrual fluid retention, but on the whole, the body is a self-regulating system as long as it is not tampered with by erratic eating habits. When you go on a strict diet, your body attempts to maintain its natural set point weight by reducing its metabolic rate. This results in a frustratingly slow weight loss if you are trying to slim quickly. After a gratifyingly rapid weight loss (mostly of fluid), you enter a plateau phase when the body interprets strict dieting as starvation and begins a sort of 'shut down' process to retain, or even regain, its set point. The resulting slow weight loss is often accompanied by an increase in appetite, constant thoughts about food and explosions of seemingly uncontrolled gorging.

You may be surprised to discover that when you actually stop dieting you are able to stabilize your weight at a level which is acceptable to you, even though you are eating three meals a day. Furthermore, if you were genuinely overweight for your height and age, you may even have managed to lose. This is because on a regular, balanced food intake your carbohydrate cravings and urges to over-eat lessen. As a result, your overall daily calorie intake is also reduced.

Bulimia sufferers also believe that purging with laxatives after a binge stops them putting on weight. However, studies show that this does not prevent calorie absorption and weight gain because food is absorbed in the small intestine before it can reach the large bowel. Any weight reduction through laxatives is due to a loss of body fluid which is eliminated (along with important salts and minerals) from the large bowel. This will be regained by drinking normally over the next few hours, but the chemical imbalance which results from the loss of minerals and electrolytes takes longer to resolve, so sufferers tend to feel weak even after they have replaced the fluid.

Self-induced vomitting is not as effective as you may think either. Sufferers frequently binge on 'fast foods', which are high in sugar and refined carbohydrates. These foods start being digested almost as soon as they enter the mouth, quickly leave the stomach, and are rapidly absorbed. Considering that binges can last anything from half an hour to several hours, it is impossible to retrieve everything that has been eaten, no matter what extremes of purging you resort to. This explains why sufferers who do not have anorexic tendencies can purge and yet stay at a normal weight, or become and remain overweight. The best way to control your weight is to stop bingeing.

If you have been maintaining an exceptionally low weight for your age, height and bone structure by long periods of fasting and/or vomitting directly after meals, however, you are bound to put on weight when you stop doing this. You may have to come to terms with the fact that nature did not intend you to have an elfin figure, and that when you eat normally your weight will creep up to a level which is probably greater than you might like it to be – or rather, than you believe fashion decrees.

Another point to consider is that height for weight charts are only a rough guide to what you should weigh. They can be misleading because it is not always easy to assess whether you have a large, medium or small frame. For example, if you have fine wrists and ankle bones you may categorize yourself as 'small framed' and believe that you should weigh half a stone less than you do. However, if you also have broad shoulders and wide hip bones it might be undesirable for you to weigh so much less.

How then do you know what is right for you? The best way is to allow your body to find its natural weight, at which point you should also be much less plagued by food cravings and urges to binge. It may be several months before your weight settles, but once you have got your eating under some sort of control it will be easier for you to think about whether setting too high a value on slimness is really worth all the misery. You could do this by listing all the pros and cons of engaging in the endless pursuit for thinness. Ideas for this are given below. You can also make a realistic assessment about how much weight you would like to lose, if any.

A list like the one below can help you to realize that what you are continuing to strive for is based on sheer fantasy and speculation. The truth of the matter is that when you eventually reach your ideal target, you will probably feel too weak and disinterested to do or enjoy any of the things you dreamed you would. Your partner is hardly going to enjoy taking you anywhere, however slim you are, if you are moody, irritable and unhappy.

Reasons for giving up dieting	Reasons against giving up
I'm always tired–my physical health is suffering.	My ego gets a lift when I lose weight.
It causes me to binge, which makes me feel that I'm losing control of my life.	My partner will enjoy taking me out if I don't look like a dumpling.
The family are suffering.	I won't dread walking into a clothes shop.
I like myself better when I'm not preoccupied about my appearance.	I'll be able to go to pop-mobility without worrying about people laughing at me.

In her book *Eating Disorders* (Routledge and Kegan Paul, 1974) Hilde Bruch discusses the devastating effects which 'making a fetish out of being thin' can have on an individual and her family. The cost in terms of serenity, chronic depression and strained relations is indeed incalculable.

Since your happiness and that of the people you are involved with is dependent on your mutual physical and emotional well-being, it is well worth taking the time to weigh up whether you are paying too heavily for your preoccupation. No matter what the slimming magazines and diet books encourage us to believe, losing weight does not help us to deal more effectively with life's challenges.

15.

A MIDDLE OF THE ROAD
APPROACH

A major self-defeating characteristic of yours may be an 'all or nothing' way of thinking. Adopting such a rigid outlook is depressingly restrictive because there is no scope for a midway approach. You may be aware that at times you see yourself as blissfully happy or deeply depressed, good or bad, fat or thin, depending on how much control you have been able to exercise over your eating. This way of thinking becomes a habit, which also affects your attitude towards dieting. You probably interpret a 'good' regime to mean never again having any of the foods you like. You may impose such strict rules on yourself that bingeing invariably occurs, either to make up for the feeling of deprivation; or so that you can indulge yourself in preparation for the forthcoming phase of starvation.

Striving to tread the middle path and to overcome the notion that certain foods are 'banned' or 'allowed' is essential if a relaxed and normal eating pattern is to be established. Try to think logically about the consequences of eating normally; for example, is one biscuit worth 80 calories really going to make you gain pounds of flab or turn you into 'a concrete blockhouse'? Reasoning with yourself in this way can help you to see that the alternative to dieting is not inevitably fatness. Stopping yourself from thinking in extremes can also prevent a session of over-eating from getting totally out of hand. For example, if after eating a bag of crisps and a couple of squares of chocolate, you feel you have done a terrible thing, and proved to yourself that you have no willpower, your guilty reactions will provoke you to feel angry, weak-willed and worthless. This distressing and self-defeating way of thinking invariably sets the stage for further panic-stricken 'all or nothing' bingeing. Panicking about the imaginary consequences of eating 'illegal' food is a recurring stumbling block for sufferers. It drives many people into full-scale bingeing and to drastic measures of weight control, so try to stem your anxiety before it gets a hold of you. The section about relaxation on page 110 may help you to control panic reactions. The books about relaxation listed on page 152 will also give you ideas on how to recognise and ease tension.

To sum up, you can prevent a moment of over-eating from snowballing into a binge, if you think about the following points.

(a) Try to take such 'slip-ups' in your stride. Remember that everyone makes them from time to time.

(b) Continue planning as constructively as possible for the rest of the day instead of telling yourself that you have completely blotted your copy book and consoling yourself with a bag of food.

(c) Try turning temporary lapses into stepping stones by looking at why you binged. Was it because of a particularly stressful situation? Were you tired or unhappy? Do you need to find some means of keeping your anxiety levels in check? How could you cope with similar events or circumstances in the future?

Changing attitudes

The following examples show how thinking in a rational way about minor setbacks can help you to fight off despair and keep on the right track.

If you find yourself thinking, 'I've binged again. This is typical. I'll never recover.' Say to yourself, 'This is a self-defeating prophecy which I can't really support since I can't predict the future with accuracy. One slip-up today doesn't mean that I can't pick up where I left off.'

In a similar way, you may think, 'Eating two biscuits just proves what a failure I am. I have no staying power.' Instead, tell yourself 'This is a sweeping and untrue statement to make about myself. If I can stick to my resolution not to binge today then I will have proved to myself that I do have staying power and that I can succeed in what I set out to do.'

Feeling at ease with the foods you fear

A practical way in which you can overcome the panic you experience when you eat 'forbidden' foods such as cakes, biscuits, bread, sweets and fatty foods, is to deliberately include a few of them in your daily diet. This requires a lot of courage, but by purposely allowing yourself to eat normal portions of the types of food usually reserved for binges, you can show yourself that you are able to exert some control over how much you eat, and that you can reduce your food cravings and desires to binge when you are not preparing for a forthcoming period of denial.

Learning to eat the foods you dread in a relaxed way is rather like learning to ride a bike. At first, you are convinced that you will topple off. However, as you go on practising, it becomes second nature and you wonder why you had any anxieties about it in the first place.

Draw up a list of everyday foods which you would like to be able to eat without panicking yourself into a binge. Start by eating one of the carbohydrates on your list which you find the least threatening, such as a slice of brown bread or a cream cracker. When you have proved to yourself that you are not going to balloon out afterwards, you can use the same approach with the rest of the items on your list. In this way you will gradually be able to challenge your irrational beliefs about forbidden foods without becoming so distressed that you launch into a frenzied binge.

The whole idea seemed a bit weird – being advised to eat the sort of things which made me feel guilty and panic-stricken. I almost believed I couldn't even look at a biscuit without turning into a dumpling – let alone digest it. I can see the value of it now, though. To begin with, I set myself small targets, such as having a taste of someone's pudding, a plain biscuit or a couple of sweets. It was very reassuring to see for myself that the effects were not at all what I thought they would be. It was no use others telling me this, however. I had to prove to myself that I could eat the same sorts of things as other people and still stay the same size.

It is important to stress that this approach is not aimed at cultivating a sweet tooth or fattening you up. It is simply a means of proving to yourself that you can eat normal amounts of so-called forbidden food without getting fat. Having established this, you can go from strength to strength, building up your confidence in your ability to control your impulses. An additional benefit of this approach will be to ease your sense of isolation. If you have been avoiding social events which centred around food, it will give you peace of mind to know that you are not going to be thrown into a panic by any foods.

> I reached a stage of refusing all invitations to go out. I was terrified someone might offer me a 'blacklisted' food – a white piece of buttered bread, an iced cake, a sausage roll or a fizzy drink. Just one nibble of these sorts of things was enough to unhinge me. I wouldn't rest until I'd got rid of it. It was only by confrontation with these sorts of food that I was eventually able to get my anxieties about them into perspective.

Constructing a personalized programme

There are various ways of planning a food programme. The food ladder shown below lists the sort of foods you might want to be able to eat with enjoyment, and above all without feeling guilty or threatened. At the bottom of the ladder should be the foods which cause you the least anxiety, and at the top those which you dread. The order you choose need have nothing to do with the calorific content of each food. Many sufferers just develop a thing about certain foods, although their energy value may be less than the foods which they are unafraid of. For example, one person may have conditioned herself to regard an ounce of cheddar cheese as a 'good' food because it is of nutritional value, and a digestive biscuit as a 'bad' food containing many fattening calories for little nutrition, whereas in fact the cheese contains more calories than the biscuit. The idea behind constructing the food ladder is to focus on the sorts of foods you would like to be able to eat normally. You must then be prepared to confront these foods regularly by including them in your normal daily or weekly food intake. For example, if milk has been on your list of forbidden foods, you could add it to tea or coffee each day. Normal amounts of staple foods such as bread, potatoes and rice could be included once or twice a day. You could eat cake, chocolates or sweets from time to time but not every day if you are worried about the effects of highly refined carbohydrates.

A food ladder

Put the foods you particularly dread at the top of the list and those which you feel least anxious about at the bottom. Work your way up the ladder item by item.

1. A portion of chips
2. A helping of cream
3. A slice of cake
4. Roast potatoes
5. A piece of chocolate
6. A portion of cheese
7. A sweet biscuit
8. A slice of bread and butter
9. A slice of bread without butter
10. A fruit-flavoured yogurt
11. A baked potato
12. A cream cracker biscuit
13. Milk in tea and coffee

When to use the ladder

Conventional meal and snack times are best. Try to be with people whose company you enjoy, and whose eating habits are reasonably standard. The advantages of this are:

(a) You will have examples of normal eating behaviour on which to model yourself. This can be particularly helpful if you are at a loss to know what constitutes an average portion, or even which sort of food to have.

(b) Having others to talk to will help to take your mind off worry and guilt about what you have eaten, thereby lessening the likelihood of panic bingeing or of making yourself sick.

Another approach aimed at helping people to regain a regular eating pattern and to have a balanced diet is that used by Andrew Carver, Senior Dietician at The Royal Edinburgh Hospital. Food is consumed in terms of portions. In addition to milk, butter or margarine, two helpings of meat, fish, egg or cheese and two helpings of vegetables, a daily total of fifteen portions is considered to be equivalent to a food intake at the lower end of normal. Once started on this regime, the number of portions is adjusted until your weight stabilises at a healthy level.

This method of dietary organisation avoids calorie counting and ensures a balanced intake of food. At the same time it

Figure 6: Portion system used by Andrew Carver

FOODS AND DRINKS TO BE TAKEN EACH DAY

¾ pint milk
½oz. butter, margarine etc.
2 helpings of the following — meat, fish, egg, cheese
2 helpings of the following – vegetables (including salad)
A total of _____ portions of the following

= 1 Portion

1 small slice bread

2 rich tea biscuits, cream crackers, ryvitas, oatcakes *etc.*

1 large digestive biscuit *etc.*

1 weetabix

1 shredded wheat

4 tablespoons cornflakes, rice krispies, puffed wheat *etc.*

1 apple, peach, pear, orange, banana

1 glass fruit juice

1 plain yoghurt

1 "diet" fruit yoghurt

1 small potato, scoop mashed potato

1 packet crisps

1 ice cream

2 tablespoons pulses (cooked)

= 2 Portions

1 roll

1 fruit yoghurt

1 chocolate biscuit e.g. – Penguin, Club *etc.*

1 croissant

1 individual fruit pie

1 individual trifle, mousse etc.

preserves a measure of protection against an unexpectedly high calorie intake and consequent weight gain which you may fear will happen when you stop purging and/or fasting.

Books containing detailed guidance on nutrition and

cooking for one person are listed in the section on further reading.

Panic attacks

You may doubt your ability to relax away your agitation when you are faced with the prospect of digesting a forbidden food. A reassuring thought, based on studies of animal and human behaviour, is that panic can only come in a wave with a limited lifespan after which it spontaneously peters out (see Figure 6). Mounting tension is very menacing and exhausting, but in order to avoid being defeated by it, try to sit it out and it will ebb away of its own accord. You will soon be able to see for yourself that what you ate did not have dire consequences for your weight or shape.

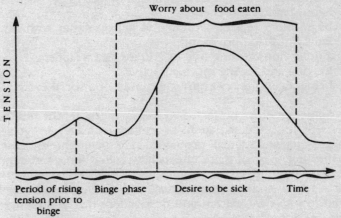

Figure 7: Diagrammatic illustration to show how panic related to eating 'Forbidden Food' spontaneously ebbs away

Imaginative tactics

If you are reluctant to launch into this approach straightaway, start by imagining yourself eating these foods. Picture yourself in a situation of having eaten a 'blacklisted' food, such as a cream cracker. Allow yourself to feel the panic and tension which arises when you eat this food, but instead of allowing it to mount, try to disperse it by whatever method of relaxation you have learnt. When you are confident that you have mastered your fears of certain foods in your imagination, you can then repeat the process for real.

Learning to feel comfortable with forbidden foods in the imagination can be valuable, providing you use it as a stepping stone to really eating the foods.

Another imaginative tactic involves focusing on the plus points of giving up bulimia. Be specific and positive, rather than vague and self-denigratory. For example, 'When I stop bingeing I'll be less of a horrible person' is not a terribly inspiring reason for stopping. Focus instead on the positive rewards of giving up, in terms of an improved quality of life. Such positive consequences would include:

greater self-discipline and respect;
improved physical health;
more money to spend on things I really want and enjoy;
more time in which to accomplish things;
extra stamina and energy;
being more relaxed and able to get on better with my family/husband/boyfriend;
a tidier house/room, free of crumbs and wrappers;
looking and feeling more attractive;
being able to really enjoy a meal out or a social event.

Some sufferers prefer to focus on the potential health hazards of bulimia, such as kidney damage, irregular heartbeats and dental problems as a deterrant to their behaviour. Fear of these effects have jolted some sufferers out of their behaviour, but they can also be counter-productive. Anxiety about damage to your health can make you feel so demoralized and despondent that you plunge into yet more bingeing.

Another tactic which has been known to put people off an unwanted behaviour is a form of self-imposed aversion therapy. This is done by dwelling on all the unpleasant aspects of your 'ritual'. When doing this, however, it is important to keep feelings about yourself and your behaviour as separate issues. Browbeating yourself for 'being disgusting' will only knock your self-esteem still further, and cause you to seek solace in a binge. Try to focus on your external behaviour alone. When the urge to binge strikes, imagine you have given in to it. Go through the bingeing ritual step by step – the stress involved in getting the food, the fear of being caught or prevented from eating what you want, the rising panic as you know you are losing control, the pain and feeling of breathlessness that goes with a distended stomach and so on, through to the process of getting rid of the food. If you concentrate on the unpleasant images connected with bingeing and purging, and then think about the benefits of alternative activities (see 'Searching for solutions' on page 107) you may well decide that you do not really want to go through with your ritual.

Guidelines for healthy eating

Try to give up dieting, even for a limited period of three or four months. Unless you resume a normal eating pattern you will go on living in fear of the unknown.

When you feel miserable about your body shape, remind yourself that no amount of dieting is going to change your bone structure, since this is determined by genetic inheritance. Remember, too, that personality and worth do not hinge on the loss or gain of a few pounds. People generally see each other as a whole, not just as a pair of fat legs or a big stomach.

Try to resist the urge to be sick after eating by involving yourself in a demanding or mentally absorbing task. Remember that sufferers who are trying to stabilize their eating often feel bloated. This is partly due to the fact that your digestive tract may not be used to processing a complete meal in one direction! Try to bear with the initial physical discomfort, and don't give in to any accompanying rising panic. After about a week of practice your gut should be back in full working order.

Try to think logically about the consequences of eating normally. It is normal to want not to be fat, but will a couple of biscuits or another helping of pudding really make you massive?

Try to avoid thinking in black or white terms, whereby you see yourself as being 'fat' or 'thin' in the same way that you binge or starve.

Try to avoid the temptation of daily weigh-ins to see if you have been 'good' or 'bad', even if this means throwing away the scales. It is typical to be sensitive to weight gain. Discovering that you have gained a couple of pounds may be enough to throw you into a depression which can only be relieved by a binge or plans to start another diet.

Try to plan three meals a day and then stick to them. You could also have a mid-morning and mid-afternoon snack. The meals you plan should provide all the essential nutrients, and a variety of tastes and textures. There is nothing quite like monotonous rounds of the same food for sparking off food cravings.

A healthy diet must be a balanced one so give up trying to live on nothing but bulky foods such as bran, muesli, raw vegetables and fruit. They fill you up quickly, and are good for you, but they do not have the same energy value as foods which contain some fat. Fat contains 9 kilocalories per gram so it is a more concentrated source of 'fuel' than proteins or carbohydrates, which contain 4 kilocalories per gram. A small amount of fat in your diet will provide you with enough 'fuel' to keep hunger at bay for at least three or four hours. This breathing space from continual hunger and thoughts of food will give you a chance to stabilize your eating and apply your mind to other interests, forgotten hobbies, and/or new ventures, all of which are important if you are to lead a more fulfilling way of life.

In the past ten to fifteen years, nutritionists and physicians have been concerned not only with the amount of fat people in the West eat, but also the type. Animal fats, which are saturated fats, were widely believed to be a cause of coronary artery disease. Fats from fish and from vegetable sources such as sunflower seeds and nuts, are polyunsaturated, and these were thought to provide protection from heart disease by reducing our blood cholesterol levels. As a result of this theory, many people adopted low fat, low cholesterol diets which were high in polyunsaturated fats. Research into these diets in more recent years, however, has failed to substantiate the claims made for the beneficial effects of polyunsaturates, and current opinion suggests that a balanced intake of fats is nutritionally desirable.

As a rough guide, your fat intake should make up not more than about one third of your total calorie intake, and about one third of the fat that you take should be polyunsaturated.

It is also worth noting that fats are an important source of vitamins A,D,E and K, and that, by allowing yourself a small amount each day, you can also keep yourself free of persistent headaches and irritability, both of which are symptoms of physiological hunger.

Try not to shy away from eating socially. It helps to see how others behave in relation to food. Being with others can also be a distraction from worrying about calories, wanting to be sick, or binge.

Try to eat at conventional mealtimes and do not skip meals, even if you are not hungry or if you have had a binge. Sticking to three meals and two snacks a day is the best way to stabilize your eating and to break the binge/purge cycle.

Try to slow down your rate of eating by resting your utensils between mouthfuls and by finishing each mouthful before starting another.

Pause at regular intervals during a meal to decide whether you still want to go on eating. Remember you do not have to finish everything on your plate if you do not want to. Practise leaving something every now and again – a few vegetables, half a potato, a bite of bread and so on.

Assert yourself when friends/family start loading up your plate with food, urging you to second helpings or persuading you to try their homemade biscuits. Have a few tactful refusals at the ready, such as, 'No thank you, I'd like to pause,' or 'I've enjoyed the meal. If I have any more I'll spoil what I've had.'

Avoid drinking a lot during mealtimes as this can make you feel bloated.

Limit the amount of food immediately available during meal or snack times by deciding how much you want and then putting the packets and cartons away. Being surrounded by open packets of food is conducive to bingeing.

If you are not sure what constitutes an average helping enlist the judgement of a friend or relative who knows about your difficulties with food. Read the instructions on the food packets, and look up recipe books, which nearly always give a guide on 'average' amounts.

Err towards smaller portions which do not make you feel over-full. You can always have a snack two or three hours later.

Make a pact to eat in one room only, preferably one

accessible to others so that temptation to binge is reduced.

Never do anything else whilst eating – or bingeing. Concentrate on tasting and savouring the food.

Cut down the amount of 'illegal' food you bring into the house and try to make the food relatively inaccessible. For example, you could place the biscuits at the top of the food cupboard rather than at eye level.

Try to live in day-tight compartments during which you set yourself realistic goals, such as 'just for this afternoon I'm not going to binge,' as opposed to 'I'm not going to binge for the rest of this month'.

Practise shopping in small quantities. Go into a general grocers with just the right amount of money to buy say a pound of apples or a couple of oranges. This way you can prove to yourself that you can walk into a shop and buy food in a controlled way.

If you have to go into a supermarket, take a hand basket rather than a trolley which you might feel that you have to fill up.

When you go shopping, take a shopping list so that you do not wander around the aisles being tempted by items of food which you don't really want or need. Take care not to shop when you feel hungry. Have a meal or snack beforehand. Go shopping at a time of the day when you feel reasonably contented. If you go at the end of a hard working day or when you are feeling down, you are much more likely to be tempted by a 'pick-me-up' of five packets of biscuits and ten loaves of bread.

Buy fresh foods which need to be prepared before being eaten instead of pre-packaged food which can be eaten on the spot.

Limit what you have to spend by leaving cheque books and banker's cards at home. Take just enough money to cover the items on your shopping list.

In the early stages of your battle against bulimia, you will find it quite hard to resist buying for a binge, so go to smaller shops rather than a supermarket. Some items may be a little more expensive and there will be less choice, but if it helps you to control your impulses it is worth the extra time and effort. It also avoids the stress of being confronted with a bewildering choice of foods.

16.

KEEPING A DIARY

The idea of a diary is to have a 'friend' in whom you can confide. Although many people dismiss writing a diary as a bit of a chore and a pointless exercise, it can be very helpful, enabling you to stabilize your eating and to sort yourself out in general. Pent-up feelings, anxieties and frustrations can be freely expressed on paper, and you can develop a greater understanding about what makes you tick, as well as monitoring your progress.

> It was encouraging to have some concrete evidence of my good days (especially if I'd been through a bad patch), and to understand myself a little better. Having successes to look back on helped to confirm in my own mind that I had what it takes to keep making strides forward.

Assemble your diary from a file of foolscap paper, rather than buying a formal book. This means that you are not restricted in your writing. You could also cover it in attractive paper or pictures to give it a more personal touch.

The next thing is to plan how to arrange it. A good idea is to divide it into sections, each one devoted to a specific problem or troubling aspect. Food will obviously be one, and ways of dealing with this have already been discussed. Other areas of discontent which can be successfully tackled with the help of a personal diary are outlined below.

Pinpointing problems

The first section of your diary could be used for pinpointing problems. Many psychologists believe that people engage in certain behaviour because it serves a purpose. In order to find out what you derive from your behaviour, use this section of your diary to note the sort of

Figure 8: Example of a Daily Food Chart

Date & Time	Activity	Mood	Hungry?	What I ate	Overall effect of my action
June 16th 9.45 a.m.	Reading the newspaper	Disappointed – expected a letter from John and it didn't arrive.	No	10 digestive biscuits, 6 slices toast & jam & butter, ⅓ pkt. cornflakes and 1½ pts milk, 2 yoghurts, ½ pkt. opal fruit sweets. 2 mugs tea. (Vomited × 4. Took 25 laxatives)	Bingeing took my mind off feeling let down, but only for a short time. I've still got to accept the fact that the letter didn't arrive. Feel more miserable than when the day began because of my lack of control.
4.15 p.m.	Shopping for mum's birthday present.	Washed out & grumpy – no idea what to buy her.	Yes (went without lunch as a penance for earlier weakness)	(In café:) 2 coffees. (On the move:) ¼lb wine gums, 1 box jelly babies, 2 kit-kats, 1 mega bar chocolate, 3 bags crisps, 2 buttered rolls, 1 pkt. maltesers, 1 can diet coke.	Total panic and self disgust. Couldn't find anywhere in the immediate vicinity to get rid of the food. Had to abandon shopping to search for a loo. Sense of failure about the entire day – failed to get mum's present and to get rid of all that chocolate.

10.30 p.m.	Plonked in a chair, supposedly watching T.V. but unable to follow the plot of the film.	Anxious & depressed. Can't stop thinking about how many calories I must have absorbed earlier on.	Don't know.	1 diet coke, 1 stick sugar free chewing gum, 1 black coffee.	Determined to be stricter with myself from now on – although my 'all' or 'nothing' attitude to food is getting me down – it's so stressful.
June 17th 8.00 a.m.	Checking my stomach & thighs for signs of weight gain.	Getting a sinking feeling about the day ahead.	Yes.	2 black coffees, 1 apple.	This is as depressing as bingeing. I'm already feeling edgy because I'm not sure how long I can keep a tight rein on my food cravings.
1.15 p.m.	Looking at the chaos in my room & worrying about this term's essay which is a week late.	Tense and guilty about my lack of interest in my studies.	Yes.	¾ loaf bread, butter, ½ jar peanut butter, 1 tin rice pudding, ¾ pkt. custard creams, 2 left over sausages, 4 bags crisps, 1 stale fruit scone, 4 mugs tea. (Vomited × 6)	This was a futile attempt to forget my worries and responsibilities. I can break the back of my essay by spending an hour or two on it now, and tidy up my room whilst listening to my new L.P. later on.
6.00 p.m.	Just back from the launderette.	Quite contented.	Yes.	1 ham omelette, tomato, slice of bread, 1 fruit yoghurt, 1 mug coffee & milk.	Great sense of achievement at having managed to eat sensibly & with restraint. More relaxed, and feel better able to take things in my stride.

circumstances and emotions which trigger a binge response.

A food record chart, similar to that shown in Figure 9, can help to get to the bottom of behaviour. In order to save writing out one sheet for each day, a week's supply could be photocopied. The cost of this will be modest compared to the expense of bingeing, and a great deal more productive.

Another means of pinpointing problems is to ask yourself a couple of questions such as:

What are the sort of events which happen just before a binge?

What are my thoughts and feelings beforehand?

What are the effects of bingeing/purging which are personally rewarding?

Finding the answers to these sorts of questions is often much more profitable than simply raking over the past to find out what initially drove you to bingeing. Although it is enlightening to discover the exact origins of your bulimia, insight alone probably will not be enough to alter the way you behave.

The value of pinpointing problems

The idea of looking at underlying reasons for your behaviour may seem a bit like opening up Pandora's box. Confronting uncomfortable feelings and thoughts is bound to be stressful, but being prepared and courageous enough to do so is an important key to recovery, along with the realization that bulimia is not solely a food and weight issue.

This may not make much sense to sufferers who are in the thick of bulimia and unable to see their behaviour as anything other than a disgusting habit which they are too weak to give up. However, as has been discussed earlier in the book, there is more to it than that, and bulimia is very often an indication that other things are wrong in a sufferer's life. It may take a while for her to recognize the connection which is why she has to analyse her feelings. For example, apart from anxieties about her appearance and/or sexual attractiveness, she may have doubts about her competence to handle responsibilities, fears of criticism resulting in lack of assertion and difficulty relating to other people, and doubts about her ability to be liked, loved, accepted and needed.

In addition, sufferers may be plagued by indecision and an overall inability to solve internal conflicts. For many this results from continual efforts to be a pleasing personality and to fit in with what everyone else wants, or what they think is expected of them. Years of doing this often result in a blurred sense of identity and difficulty in determining what one really wants out of life.

Another background feature of bulimia may be difficulty in expressing feelings. For example, anger and resentment felt by sufferers towards their family or friends may run deep, yet, because of continual fear of disapproval, they dare not allow their true emotions to surface. Feelings which are too painful to confront and deal with get pushed underground where they fester and may lead to depression. The slough of despond into which depressed people so readily fall is fertile ground for addictions to take root in. We have already seen that compulsive thoughts about food and weight serve as distractions for bulimia sufferers.

> Food has become my only source of satisfaction and solace ...

> It's all I look forward to at the end of the day ... it gives me a flicker of comfort and is the only means I have of forgetting all my problems

Understanding that bulimia can mask a diversity of interwoven problems helps a sufferer to look beyond the food and weight issues. Such insight can be very reassuring to people who feared they might be going off the rails about food. Once they have faced up to the underlying problems, they can begin to look for less destructive means of coping with them.

If you cannot work out what it is that makes you binge, try quizzing yourself on a few of the following questions.

Is bingeing a way of avoiding:

(a) upsetting thoughts about yourself or others;
(b) unhappy moods;
(c) empty hours ahead when you have nothing in particular to do;
(d) other people (sexual or emotional entanglements)?

Is it a means of:

(a) releasing tension;

(b) feeling self-reliant;

(c) calming yourself down – your ever-available 'tranquillizer';

(d) diverting yourself from something you don't want to knuckle down to, such as studying, tidying up a room, writing a letter;

(e) having a break from the tormented existence of dieting;

(f) getting back at people who have hurt you;

(g) getting special attention or consideration from others;

(h) excitement – of getting an illicit feeling of pleasure because you are getting away with something you should not be doing?

Does purging serve as:

(a) a punishment for being so weak-willed;

(b) a cleansing feeling;

(c) an immense relief, which you look forward to when you are bingeing

(d) a reassurance – at the end of the day you still have the upper hand over your weight problem;

(e) a way of getting rid of aggressive feelings?

Identifying what it is you get from your behaviour that is personally rewarding or useful, will make it easier to work out alternative, less destructive, means of obtaining the same effects.

Searching for solutions

A second section of your diary could be allocated to searching for solutions to your difficulties. Even if you do not feel ready or prepared to acknowledge the problems that lead you to binge, you can still work on practical ways of interrupting the binge/purge cycle. The second section of your diary could therefore concentrate on ways of avoiding bingeing. A good idea is to write out a list of alternative activities. These obviously will not be an exact substitute for eating, but they will help you to get back into the mainstream of life and enable you to cope more effectively.

It is easy to talk about alternatives to bingeing, and even to list them, but when it comes to the crunch of having to say 'no' to cravings for food, it is another story. Imagination, effort and a lot of self-discipline are needed to keep fighting back on the road to recovery. As daunting and tedious as this may seem, and however much you have to force yourself to try an alternative, your efforts will boost your morale and give you the stamina to stay the course.

It is a good idea to include a wide range of activities which allow for a variation in mood. It is also important to ensure that the rather run-of-the-mill sorts of activities are mixed with more extravagent ones which involve spending money. The following example illustrates the variety to aim for.

Everyday things which are enjoyable and which can be carried out easily and immediately
Phoning a friend.
Knitting.
Watching television.
Wallowing in a bubble bath.
Browsing through a photo album.
Curling up in a chair with a good book.
Reading a glossy magazine.
Experimenting with make-up.
Tending the indoor plants.
Listening to a record.
Fifteen minutes of relaxation.
Going for a run.

Things which promote a sense of achievement
Tidying the bedroom drawers.
Writing letters.
Updating the address book.
Taking up a new hobby.
Mending clothes.
Doing the ironing.

Special rewards
Having a new hair style.
Buying a new dress or jumper.
Getting theatre or cinema tickets.
Having a long lie-in.
Treating yourself to a bunch of flowers or a pot plant.

The list of possible rewards and alternatives is of course endless. You can make them as invigorating, intellectually stimulating, adventurous or creative as you want them to be. The point to remember is that if one strategy fails you can always try another. It may seem a waste of time to write out a list, but if you're someone who experiences a blind vacancy of mind when the urge to binge strikes, having a written list to hand will undoubtedly be of benefit. It is an effective way of preparing for times of temptation, and preparation of any sort inevitably requires a bit of effort.

A list can help in various ways.

1. It can help you to stall a binge, if you say, for example, 'Rather than binge over the next hour I could read the newspaper over a leisurely cup of coffee.'
2. It can help you to get back into the mainstream of life. Hard or unstimulating work forms the core of most people's day. Tidying, sorting, writing difficult letters or essays may not be the world's most exciting tasks, but by buckling down to them and accepting them as part and parcel of life, you can begin to lead a normal life and, above all, build up a sense of personal worth.
3. It can cut down the stress in your life. Facing up to the demands mentioned above prevents them from turning into ogres. Tension and apprehension can build up in people who continually 'put off until tomorrow what may be done today', especially if there are deadlines to be met. If a thing has to be done, do it now, instead of trying to blot it out with a binge.
4. It can help you to overcome difficult moments related to eating. Sensations of fullness often drive individuals to panic binge or to make themselves sick. A list of enjoyable or constructive things to do will help to channel your thoughts away from worrying about what you have just eaten.
5. Apart from helping to avoid bingeing, a list of alternatives teaches the value of looking after yourself in an appropriate way and at relevant times, regardless of weight or shape.

As one sufferer explains:

I've learnt to bow to the inevitable. I'm never going to have a pencil-thin waist or skinny thighs. My body shape is not what I would call ideal, but I've come to appreciate it's at least working. These days I try to concentrate on making the best of what I've got, by keeping healthy, eating properly and keeping my weight stable with the help of some exercise.

Feeling good about yourself in this way raises your sense of self-worth, which in turn assists relationships with others. You can begin to appreciate your good points, instead of always focusing on the real or imaginary 'bad' ones, and accept compliments in the spirit in which they were intended.

I was the archetypal 'good girl', yet I could only see 'bad' in myself. This feeling of being 'no good' colours my view of everything. If someone says something nice about me I instantly dismiss it as an idle compliment.

6. A list helps you to structure time. Unplanned lulls during a normally busy day can cause a panic about what to do and especially how to cope with being alone. Instead of drifting aimlessly and trying to get rid of that stressful 'in limbo' sensation by bingeing, look down your list of alternatives for something which will make spare time enjoyable.

If nothing appeals, it is worth trying something constructive which will promote a rewarding sense of achievement.

Some of my most intense food cravings would strike, not when I was absorbed in a task of some sort, but when I was moping about. Doing something, whether it was scrubbing the kitchen floor or frisking around to my favourite record, stopped me from dwelling on thoughts of food.

7. You can learn to slow down the tempo of life. The value of keeping stimulated and occupied as a deterrent to bingeing has been emphasized, but time should also be set aside for some rest and relaxation. Although a certain amount of stress is necessary and healthy because it motivates people to accomplish things which make them feel good, life can seem unmanageable if the accent is totally on keeping busy. Everyone needs to have a break from the demands of their work, surroundings and family in order to keep in touch with

themselves. Sufferers from bulimia often fail to do this in a constructive way. They often cannot tolerate their own company and end up bingeing as a means of getting away from themselves and others.

All I look forward to at the end of a day is collapsing with a bag of food. I know it's self-indulgent but it's the only way I can switch off one hundred per cent. I know food isn't going to make any demands on me, and it's always around when I need it.

The importance of relaxing has already been mentioned in connection with learning to eat the foods you fear. It is one of the best ways to keep stress in check.

Relaxation

People often say that they 'just can't relax', when in fact they have never really tried. Others ask 'Why bother – how exactly does relaxation help?' It helps in the following ways.

1. It gives you a mental break from the demands being made upon you.
2. It relieves you of some of the anxiety and physical tension which drives you to bingeing.
3. It sets the right tone for the rest of the day.

After twenty or thirty minutes of relaxation I feel calm and much more able to take things in my stride.

There are many forms of relaxation, ranging from the ancient traditions of yoga and meditation to more modern methods such as The Alexander Technique, Autogenic Training, and Biofeedback.

You can train yourself to relax by going to classes, or by learning from tapes and books at home.

Classes are a good way of meeting other people. You can find out about them from local newspapers; shop window advertisements, particularly newsagents; libraries; friends and neighbours; the Citizens Advice Bureaux.

Tapes have the advantage of enabling you to practise whenever you want in the seclusion of your own home. Relaxation tapes can be bought, or made by a friend or relative. A charity called 'Relaxation for Living' (the address is given on page 147) produces lots of helpful leaflets and a comprehensive booklist, and organizes countrywide classes and correspondence courses to help people learn to relax.

The following guidelines may be useful if you want to practise your own form of relaxation.

Preparatory steps
1. Get into the habit of practising for twenty or thirty minutes each day.
2. Choose a time of day in which you are unlikely to be disturbed.
3. Minimize distractions by closing windows and doors.
4. Wear comfortable, loose but warm clothing.
5. Lie flat on your back with your legs straight out in front and your feet loosely together. Keep your arms by your sides and your hands unclenched, with the palms facing upwards, close your eyes.

Breathing
Many relaxation techniques focus on controlled breathing. You can begin to learn this alone at any time, anywhere.

1. Breathe deeply, slowly and evenly to a count of four or five, in through your nose and out through your mouth.
2. With each breath out, say the word 'relax'.
3. Think of your mind as a cluttered room. Carefully vacuum out all the irritations, resentments, worry, disappointments and frustrations of the past hours, days, and weeks.
4. Picture a scene or situation which induces a feeling of contentment and calm. It might be a peaceful country setting, a calm sea, or a beach on an idyllic tropical island.

Relaxing tension
With a relaxed frame of mind, you can learn to recognize tension in your body. Do this by practising a simple clenching and relaxing of the muscles.

1. Starting with your toes, clench them tight, and tighter still. Hold for a count of five, noticing the tension, and then slowly let go.

2. Using this technique, work systematically up your body. Tense your calves, thighs and buttocks by pulling your legs together, and then relax. Tense the muscles in your stomach as if you are about to be punched. Relax. Take a deep breath to tighten the chest muscles then exhale to relax them. Then start on your arms. Make a fist and then relax your fingers. Bend your elbow as firmly as possibly to tense your forearm and then relax. Press your head backwards to tighten your neck and then relax. Frown hard and relax. Push your tongue up against the roof of your mouth and then relax. Wrinkle up your nose and screw your eyes up tightly and then relax. At each stage, try to notice the difference between the loose floppy state of relaxation and the state of tension.

3. Finally, imagine your body as a set of taut strings which are becoming slacker and slacker with every breath out. Continue to regulate your breathing. Breathe deeply, slowly and gently. Focusing your attention on breathing will enhance the overall calming effect of relaxation.

With practice, you will soon come to know the difference between being unnecessarily keyed up and suitably relaxed. The ultimate aim should be to integrate whichever technique you choose into your daily life, so that you are relaxed in whatever you do, whether it is sitting at an office desk, having a meal, or feeling at a loose end.

Setting Goals

Another section of your diary could be set aside for 'goal-keeping'. Setting goals can enable you to stabilize your eating and to develop a new sense of direction and purpose about life, but make sure you keep them realistic. Setting your expectations too high may cause you to feel hopelessly inadequate when goals are not achieved. Try to take each morning, afternoon, and evening a step at a time. This makes it much easier to get through the day without bingeing. It would be unrealistic for a person who has been bingeing and making herself sick three or four times a day to expect to snap out of her behaviour overnight. A more realistic approach would be to try to halve the frequency of her bingeing over a fortnight, and to cut it down still further over the following two weeks. At the same time, she could be experimenting with alternative strategies which will help to fill the vacuum left by not bingeing.

Some general tips for goal-keeping are summarized below.

1. Try to assess the way you live now.
2. Work out personal priorities based on what you want. (People who learn to fulfill their own needs first find that their contentment reverberates on to others.)
3. List the things you would like to change and/or want to achieve in terms of:
   (a) relationships;
   (b) studies or career;
4. Separate goals into short, medium and long-term aims so that you do not nurture unrealistic ambitions.
5. Avoid saying 'I must', 'I will', 'I should'. Go for a more relaxed approach that can be modified to suit changing circumstances, such as, 'I would like', 'I want to try', 'I could'.
6. Be prepared to strike a balance between what you would like to do and what is actually possible.
7. Go over your list of goals every so often. Where some doors close others will open and you may have to adjust your sights accordingly.
8. Whatever goals you choose to set yourself, it is important to remember that everything has a small beginning. However small and infrequent your experiences of success are, they will make a more lasting impact on your overall well-being, than aiming for an overnight cure.

Within the goal-setting context there are four states which are particularly relevant to women with bulimia. These are depression, perfectionism, lack of assertiveness and the problem of loneliness. How these affect your life, and how you can deal with them, is discussed in the next chapters.

17.

DEALING WITH DEPRESSION

If you feel that depression is an underlying cause for your eating problem, mention this to your doctor or therapist.

Depression can show itself in any of the following ways:

(a) feelings of total despair/failure/hopelessness and helplessness;
(b) disinterest in close relationships, family or friends;
(c) disinterest in hobbies and poor concentration;
(d) feelings of guilt and unworthiness;
(e) feelings of indecision and isolation.

Physical symptoms can include:
(a) overeating, particularly if you are very anxious;
(b) frequent headaches;
(c) tearfulness;
(d) restlessness;
(e) sleeplessness, yet always feeling tired.

How depression starts

There are three main types of depression. Endogenous depression comes right out of the blue and there often seems to be no reason for it. Secondary depression results from a physical illness of viral origin, such as infective hepatitis (an infected liver), flu, shingles, or glandular fever. The third form, reactive depression, is the most common. It follows a loss such as a death in the family, a broken love affair, the loss of a cherished object, and getting married or having children, both of which can make people feel that they have lost their freedom.

People differ over how long it takes to come to terms

with their loss, but those who do not complete the mourning process may become chronically depressed later on in life. They may have overcome the initial stages of numbness and disbelief but failed to pass through the stages of acceptance and adjustment. Instead they continue to yearn and emotionally search for what is lost. Feelings of sadness, guilt and anger – emotions which are all part of the mourning process – intensify and deepen, propelling them into gloom and despair. Everything around them becomes a sob story. They reflect a lot on the past, fear the future, become very irritable and fail to see any meaning in life or good in themselves.

Depression is thought to be worse for you if you lack a close and loving relationship with either a husband or boyfriend, and this is often the case for bulimia sufferers. Secrecy, feelings of unworthiness, shame about your eating habits, and intense self-dislike make it difficult to establish and maintain confiding relationships, and this increases the sufferer's sense of isolation. Eventually, depression can become a way of life and in some instances serves a useful purpose. People may treat you with kid gloves so as not to hurt your feelings, or try to shield you from the reality of life in case you become worse. In effect, it enables you to escape responsibilities. This may sound fine but, as stated earlier in the book, the only way to get what you want out of life and overcome unwanted behaviour of any sort is to take full charge of yourself.

How to deal with depression

Making a conscious decision to stop bingeing is something you alone must do, since no one can do it for you, but as mentioned earlier, it may unmask or trigger feelings of depression.

> Bingeing had become such an integral part of my life. Without it I seemed to fall into a vacuum ... a pit of black despair.

When the bingeing subsides and troubling emotions begin to surface, guard against trying to soldier on without support 'so as not to bother others'. This may seem praiseworthy at first sight, but it can backfire, driving you deeper into despair and feelings of being all alone. Do try talking it through with other people. This is one of the most helpful ways to combat a sense of desolation and despondency.

> My sister and boyfriend spurred me on during the bleak times. When I felt recovery was an impossibility it was a great help to have someone to tell me, 'You can do it.' I know now that problems can't be solved by eating. Now, whenever I have an 'off day', I try to talk to someone about it, rather than burying my head in the biscuit barrel.

These tips may help you to cope with your depression.

1. Remember that depression is an essentially normal response to loss. Everyone goes through emotional cycles of ups and downs, admittedly in varying degrees of intensity depending on the nature of the loss. They are a part of life, and without the 'lows', we would not be able to appreciate the happier times.
2. The same can be said of disappointments and failures. Everyone experiences them from time to time, and your morale inevitably takes a knock, but it is important not to let your spirit be broken by them. Have faith in yourself to rise above them and aim to make a go of any future opportunities that come your way.
3. Guard against cocooning yourself in self pity. It will turn molehills into mountains and keep you in the clutches of apathy and hopelessness.
4. Try a method of relaxation (see page 110).
5. The book list on page 153 describes some books that deal more fully with the problems of depression.
6. If you visit a doctor, and anti-depressant treatment is prescribed, it may take several weeks to have a beneficial effect. It is essential to keep taking medication until the doctor stops it. Remember to report any unpleasant side effects.

Changing your view

A number of doctors now see the value of encouraging depressed individuals to alter pessimistic thought patterns which lead to destructive feelings and behaviour. Adopting a bleak outlook on life drains you of a lot of emotional energy which could be directed towards other activities. Studies have shown that when negative assumptions and attitudes are viewed from a more positive angle, your interpretation of life's events and circumstances can alter considerably for the better. Trying to restructure your negative ways of thinking may sound like a tall order, particularly if you feel so depressed that you cannot be bothered with anything. However, it is worth trying to develop the right mental weapons to combat the feelings of doom, self-blame and despair which probably overshadow you. If you can do this it also means that you do not have to succumb to depression as a passive victim, whereby you feel powerless to do anything to help yourself. The examples below show that negative emotions can be sparked off not so much by an event as by *how* you see the event. Learning to recognize and then challenge your faulty vision is an effective way of by-passing blind alleys of despair.

The following examples illustrate how irrational ideas can be countered by rational thoughts.

(a) 'I can't change; I'm bound to make a hash of it if I even try. It's best to keep going the way I am.'
(b) 'There's always an element of risk in a bid to solve problems. If I carefully weigh up the pros and cons of what I do I can lessen the risks involved. This would be better than staying stuck in a rut.'

(a) 'I must be loved and accepted by everyone.'
(b) 'This is unrealistic – nobody can please everyone.'

(a) 'I've been shaped by the past. It's too late to change.'
(b) 'I'm in charge of my own life now. My feelings are mine alone. I am able to grow at my own pace and in whichever way I choose.'

(a) 'I think everything is going to be terrible.'
(b) 'Life is full of rough and smooth paths. I can't predict the future with accuracy. It might not be as bad as I imagine it will be.

If you tend to think in a negative way, you may be interested to find out more about this method of helping yourself. A book which includes more detailed explanations about 'The Cognitive Theory' is recommended on page 153.

You could try to change your negative thinking patterns in the following ways.

1. Try to become more aware of what you are thinking.
2. Try showing yourself that some of your thoughts are inaccurate and misconceived.
3. Try to challenge these inaccurate and often pessimistic thoughts with ones which are nearer to the truth and geared for positive action.
4. Keep an informal record, in a diary or notebook, of two or three fairly typical negative thoughts which regularly come to your conscious mind, especially when you are depressed.
5. Over a few days try to think about these thoughts in a way that is not biased by personal emotions or preconceptions. Ask yourself some of the following questions to help counteract your view of yourself and the world.

   (i) Is there any hard evidence to support your view of yourself / the world / other people?
   (ii) When terrible things happen does this automatically mean that other people are terrible?
   (iii) Are other people really exempt from the sort of trials and difficulties you are experiencing?
   (iv) Are others really having an easier time?
   (v) Don't others sometimes have it worse?
   (vi) Is life going to come to an end because of what has happened?
   (vii) Are you going to be dominated by the past or are you going to break free of it and exercise the right to please yourself?
   (viii) Do others really expect so much from you or are you expecting too much from yourself?
   (ix) Are you taking a balanced view of yourself? Are you recognizing your assets and not just focusing on your real or imagined shortcomings?
   (x) Are your thoughts really facts, or just misunderstood beliefs or assumptions?

Changing your way of thinking can sound quite simple

but when you first start trying to do this, rational answers may not come to mind immediately or easily. This is the reason for suggesting that you initially focus on just two or three typically negative and frequently recurring thoughts. When you have been able to get these into perspective you can go on to identify a few others. The more you test yourself in this way, the more natural the process becomes and the greater your resilience to self-defeating beliefs.

Pessimistic predictions can also be put to the test in a practical way. Supposing, for example, you tell yourself 'I'm never going to manage to get through this evening without bingeing'. You can put this self-defeating assumption to the test by seeing if you can go for the next fifteen to thirty minutes without bingeing. Draw up a timetable of hourly slots in which you write down the alternatives to bingeing which you intend to accomplish. By building on a series of small successes, you can prove to yourself that you are in control of what you do, as opposed to 'feeling programmed to eat.'

Depression and the pre-menstrual syndrome

Many women are aware that a week to ten days before a period they feel an increased sense of anxiety coupled with depression, lethargy, irritability and general bloatedness. In addition, their eating goes awry. They crave high calorie foods such as cream-filled cakes, doughnuts, sweets and chips. An alteration in the hormone balance which causes the blood sugar levels to fall, and a shortage of essential fatty acids are thought to be the cause of the trouble. Although pre-menstrual symptoms usually clear up when the period begins, if you feel they contribute significantly to your problems with food, you could keep a record of them to show your doctor. When the pre-menstrual symptoms begin, make a note of the date, and what form the symptoms take. Keep a daily record until the end of your period, noting down how long the pre-menstrual symptoms and the period last. Keep a record of your menstrual cycle for three or four months and then show it to your doctor.

If your doctor thinks pre-menstrual syndrome is a significant problem, he or she may suggest that you take diuretic pills which will relieve the bloatedness caused by

pre-menstrual fluid retention. Symptoms should not, however, be overplayed simply to obtain diuretics in the mis-
taken belief that these will provide an effortless way to lose
weight. When used frequently and for the wrong reasons,
dependency tends to develop, resulting in dehydration and
upsets in the chemical composition of the blood similar to
those caused by laxative abuse. A course of vitamin B_6 or
evening primrose oil may also be prescribed to help correct the efficiency with which the body tissue makes use of
essential fatty acids.

You can relieve some of the symptoms yourself in the
following ways.

1. Try some form of relaxation, such as yoga or medita-
    tion.
2. Make sure that you do not go for more than three
    hours without a snack. This will help to prevent your
    blood sugar level falling too low and sparking off car-
    bohydrate cravings.
3. Learn more about the syndrome. There are a number
    of books on the market which deal specifically with
    methods of self-help for the pre-menstrual syndrome,
    some of which are listed on page 154.
4. Make sure that you get enough sleep. Many women
    find that they feel extra tired before a period.
    Tiredness can lower your resistance to the daily stress-
    es of life, and make you more vulnerable to bingeing.
5. Do not panic about putting on weight; this is caused
    by fluid retention and will disappear when your period
    starts.
6. Take a bit of trouble with your appearance. Clean hair
    and clothes and a touch of make-up can do a lot to
    keep you from getting too down in the dumps. You
    may feel awful, but you will feel even worse if you
    think you look awful too.
7. Remember that pre-menstrual symptoms are
    experienced by hundreds of women every month. Just
    being aware of the cause of your symptoms is often a
    great help in relieving you of anxiety. You are not
    taking a turn for the worse when they arise. They are
    part of a normal physiological process, and are
    temporary.

18.

DEALING WITH PERFECTIONISM

A close look at perfectionism shows just how much of a negative impact it can make on your life and why it is worth trying to curtail it.

> Whatever I do, and however well people say I've done something, this little voice pipes up, 'There's always room for improvement.' I'm always struggling to reach the top of the mountain, and the fact that I never quite get there often makes life seem so pointless.

Perfectionism guarantees failure. It can drive you to try to move heaven and earth, and leave you feeling so demoralized and hesitant when you 'fail', that a sort of paralysis eventually sets in. Fears of looking silly and being criticized or rejected if you do not quite make the grade can undermine your confidence so much that you never try anything new. You may feel that it is not worth doing anything unless you can get it exactly right.

Despite this rather gloomy picture of perfectionism, a reassuring thought is that all human beings have the potential to change their way of thinking and to see things from several angles.

In the last chapter, it was explained that by challenging inaccurate thoughts with those which are nearer to the truth, you can bring a touch of realism to distorted impressions of yourself and the world. The same approach can be used to combat perfectionism if it has a negative effect on you.

For example, a person who tends to be a perfectionist will probably think 'I must be well thought of by everyone.

I must be perfectly competent and successful in everything I set out to do. Unless something shows promising signs of turning out just right I may as well give up.'

You can challenge such thoughts by saying, 'Am I expecting myself to be superhuman? I may not be perfect, but does this mean I have no right to do things for the sheer pleasure and fun of doing them? Do I expect the same sort of performance from others as I inflict on myself? Am I using double standards?'

By asking yourself these sorts of questions you can keep a sense of proportion about your perceived shortcomings, and free yourself from the fears, self-condemnation and frustration which perfectionism breeds. You can accept that, like everyone else, you have your limitations. Furthermore, you will feel better placed to tackle remaining areas of discontent which may have held you back from joining in the rough and tumble of life.

Helpful hints

Give up comparing your social status, material possessions, or personal appearance with other people's. Aim to build up a sense of your own value that does not rely upon success or other people's approval.

When things do not work out quite as you expected them to, do not write yourself off as a failure.

19.

ASSERTING YOURSELF

Everyone saw me as someone with a permanently sunny
disposition, full of bounce and always ready to help, no matter
how personally inconvenient. I was always attuned to the
needs of those around me. I felt obliged to make them happy. I
shrank from the idea of having to lean on anyone, and
arguments were avoided at all costs. The price for this mask of
charm and compliance turned out to be a simmering inner fury
and rebellion. Eating helped to muffle these feelings which I
just couldn't handle.

If you suffer from bulimia the chances are that you will
identify quite closely with the above quotation. You may
be aware that you also have great difficulty putting your
own needs before those of others, and that as a result, your
self-esteem and sense of integrity get knocked to pieces. In
addition, you may feel that you have no right to stand up to
anyone in authority, to make demands, or to let others
down. Your desire for approval may be so intense that you
put up with things you do not like rather than making a
scene or rocking the boat. The result is that you continue to
feel manipulated and trampled upon, and relationships
break down when these feelings erupt in sulks or rages.
Psychologists tell us that keeping our emotions pent up
often causes them to emerge in a destructive sideways
fashion. Anger, for example, is a normal human emotion
but many women are afraid to admit to it for fear of being
labelled 'unfeminine' or, worse still, 'neurotic'. Yet unless it
is acknowledged and properly aired it is likely to be turned
inwards, leaving you full of self-contempt and dislike.
Sorrow and heartache which you have never talked about

or cried over can cause you to feel uneasy and threatened about getting close to others for fear of revealing yourself. In resisting closeness you can become increasingly isolated and thus the stage may be set for binge eating, heavy drinking, depression, and so forth.

Learning to assert yourself

'Self assertion' has received a lot of publicity in recent years. Classes have sprung up throughout the country to help people to articulate their thoughts and needs in a way which is not abrasive, pushy, or manipulative. If you are aware that you have difficulty expressing yourself and your needs in an appropriate way you might find a course or a book (see page 154) on assertiveness of enormous value in enabling you to feel better about yourself, and to realize that you do not have to live your life through the eyes of others in order to be appreciated and loved. In the long run, letting others know where you stand and being true to yourself is much better for establishing satisfactory personal relationships and for increasing your chances for getting what you want out of life.

> I read a sort of self-help book on self-assertion and found it helped both my eating and my depression. All my life I felt as if I had been shuffled around by other people. It helped me to realize that in subtle and gentle ways I can look after my own interests and just be me.

Focusing on feelings

It is easy to talk about the importance of asserting ourselves and expressing our feelings directly, but if you suffer from bulimia you may have lost touch with many things in life, including your feelings. Furthermore, if you have been brought up to believe it is embarrassing or feeble to say what you feel, it can be very difficult to cast aside your inhibitions. Even finding the right words to describe what you feel can become a problem if you are so unused to doing it.

When you are talking about your feelings, try to get beyond superficial thoughts and identify what you really feel. There is a subtle but important difference between expressing your feelings and merely saying what you think of someone. Look at these two statements.

I think you just like to poke fun at me.

I feel hurt and angry because when I tripped up you just stood and laughed at me instead of helping me to my feet.

The first statement is vague and non-specific and much more likely to put the person you are talking to on the defensive. The second statement states quite clearly why you are upset and opens the way for a discussion, explanation, or apology. The same applies to these two statements.

I think you don't care about me anymore.

I feel hurt and resentful that you went drinking with your friends instead of taking me out on my birthday like you normally do.

The first statement is simply a vague criticism. The second one provides the other person with an immediate awareness of how you feel, and why, and is much more likely to initiate a discussion.

Of course, it is not always easy in the heat of the moment to separate your thoughts and feelings, particularly if you are not used to doing so.

A good way to become familiar with expressing your feelings is to practise. There may be someone in your family or at work, such as your boss, your partner, your mother, or a friend, with whom you would like to communicate in a more genuine way. Imagine a typical conversation which you might have with them. Think of the sort of statements you tend to make. How many of them really convey what you feel?

If you find that you are literally lost for words when you try to describe your feelings, sit down with a dictionary and make a list of all the enjoyable and unpleasant feelings you think you might experience.

Here is an example to start you off.

Positive feelings	Negative feelings
Amazed	Afraid
Astonished	Angry
Appreciation	Blue

Positive feelings	**Negative feelings**
Calm	Cross
Comfortable	Disappointed
Delighted	Depressed
Excited	Frustrated
Free	Hate
Happy	Guilty
Loving	Irritated
Secure	Sad
Warm	Jealous
Thankful	Resentful

So, to re-cap, aim to express your feelings as clearly as possible and remember to be specific when you are complaining about a person's behaviour. Describe exactly what it is that upsets you, rather than generalizing and making personal critiscisms. Avoid personal insults at all costs. These can rile people to the extent that they respond to your comments with rage, and your original complaint will be overlooked.

You can also practise asking for specific changes in a person's behaviour. The following examples give you an idea of how to do this.

For the past week you've come home and just fallen asleep in front of the television. I enjoy going out once in a while and would like it if we could set aside an evening next week, say Friday, to see a film or eat out.

I'm angry that I had to get the bus to my evening class because you weren't home when you said you would be. I'd like it if you could fix a different evening to go drinking with your friends so that I could have the car when I need it.

Some hints on self-assertion

1. Choose your time carefully. Don't make a complaint to someone who has just got home after a busy day or who is feeling a bit depressed or out of sorts. You are unlikely to get the response that you want.
2. Remember to express your good feelings as well as your negative ones. You might brighten up someone else's day and spread some happiness.

3. Failing to hit it off with everyone is not a personal failing, it is a facet of human nature. Encountering some form of rejection is an everyday experience for everyone. It does not mean that the world rejects you.

4. Everyone feels hostile at times and has hurt, angry feelings. It does not mean you are a wicked person, mentally unstable or odd. In fact, anger, if appropriately chanelled, can be a very positive force. It can be sweated away in a gym, dusted away with the housework, or punched away on a pillow. Expressing it need not involve direct confrontation with the person who caused you to feel angry, and it is worth finding a physical outlet for it that is going to provide you with a healthy sense of accomplishment, rather than a guilty conscience.

5. Do not be afraid of asking others for help when you need it. This can be a problem if you have a tendency to worry a lot about putting people out, or feel unworthy of favours. Remember that most people derive pleasure and satisfaction from helping others, and you might be making someone else feel good by requesting their help.

6. Be direct when making a request, and if it is agreed to, guard against repeatedly asking the person if they are 'sure it's really OK'. Here is an example of a straightforward request: 'Hello Jane, it's Debbie, please could I have a lift tomorrow morning?' Avoid giving detailed explanations as to why you are having to ask a favour. A brief one should be enough, such as, 'My car's going into the garage for an overhaul.' Express your gratitude in a simple statement, such as, 'Thanks, I'm very grateful', and avoid giving a string of promises about how you intend to re-pay your debt. It can be irritating and embarrassing for the other person who may already have assumed that you would be happy to return the favour in a reverse situation.

7. It is awkward when you have to turn down requests from other people, but it inevitably happens from time to time. Try giving honest refusals in response to demands. Do not feel you have to spin a story or

provide a series of excuses for being unable to meet someone's needs. For example, if you are asked to babysit on a night when you have arranged to go out, just say, 'I'm sorry I can't, I've arranged to go out on Thursday.' A polite refusal followed by a brief explanation should be enough. This allows the person making the request to get on with the job of finding someone else to help her out, and will make you feel less guilt-ridden than if you launch into a string of apologies and excuses along the lines of, 'I'm so sorry ... if only I'd known sooner ... I would change my arrangements if I could but Jane doesn't have a 'phone ...' and so on.

8. Saying calmly what you want, feel or need is a much more productive way to communicate, and is less likely to infuriate others, than launching into a binge, erupting with rage or sulking. For example, if someone says something teasing or unkind about you, ask them to explain exactly what they meant and why.

9. If your love life leaves much to be desired, take the initiative of treating yourself to a book on the subject of lovemaking skills, sexual behaviour and birth control. It helps to know what other people get up to, and you may acquire a clearer understanding about some of your own attitudes to sex. Books offer information and advice, but are not always sufficient if you are experiencing practical difficulties. In this case, think about obtaining help from a trained counsellor (see pages 145–6 for some addresses). The quickest way for a sex problem to get worse and turn into a nagging stress is for you to silently worry about it. Furthermore, an unhappy sex life can put great strain on a relationship. Alternative sources of help might be your family doctor or your family planning clinic.

10. Another area of discontent and therefore stress might be your job. If it is getting you down, do not feel locked in it. Decide whether you want the same job but in another company, or a different scene altogether. Write to other places that interest you, and look in newspapers, job centres, and public libraries for training opportunities. Also, keep a look out for agencies offering vocational guidance.

11. Remember that life is meant to be enjoyed rather than endured like some sort of prison sentence. Be a friend to yourself and experience pleasures which you have previously denied yourself. Cast aside thoughts of being undeserving, or not worthwhile as you go down your list of alternatives to bingeing (see page 107). Something will appeal to you as being just right for the mood you are in.

20.

OVERCOMING LONELINESS

Human beings need more than just calories, water, light and oxygen. They need friends for their emotional well-being and without close, confiding bonds, feelings of deadness and emptiness soon set in. Many bulimia sufferers are basically lonely and lack true companionship, as the following examples show.

> I started going to pieces. Whereas before I'd always been as bright as silver, I couldn't be bothered with anything. My sense of humour vanished, as did my sense of belonging. The more I retreated into myself, the more I depended on food for everything. Making proper contact with people became too much of an effort, yet at the same time I was so frightened of myself, my own company, and of being alone.

> Bingeing (on food and drink) became the highlight of my day. I'd stagger home after work under a mountain of groceries to my dreary little hide-away bed-sit. then I'd sit and eat until I felt too stuffed to want anything, other than to be sick.

If you lack close, warm relationships, you can quickly come to feel deprived. In your deprivation you feel depressed and rejected, and it is hard to make any sense of life. Over-indulging your physical needs, whether it is by binge-eating, taking drugs or drinking too much, can then become a way of compensating for the things you lack, and in particular, for easing the ache of loneliness. The snag with using these forms of compensation is that when the 'high' and the excitement wears off, you are back to the 'low' of feeling lonely. Also, you may have looked to casual sex as a substitute for a proper relationship, and then found that it is only an imitation of the warmth and loving closeness experienced between people who genuinely care for each other. So you remain caught in your loneliness.

Alternatively, you may have gone a stage beyond using your behaviour as a compensation or painkiller. It may have become an established substitute for your need for closeness and love. You may have become so adjusted to your lack of intimacy with other people that when you are confronted with opportunities for friendship, you become anxious and frightened. It is rather like the effect sunlight has on the eyes of a person who has been enclosed in a dark room; on first exposure they ache.

Problems with eating, coupled with a deep sense of inadequacy, obviously make it very difficult to form and keep close friendships. You may feel unsure of the value of anything you do, of your identity, of trusting yourself or others. A foolproof method of increasing your self-esteem is to build a few bridges and knock down some barriers. Other people can help you to get a clearer picture of who you are and to value what you do. Their views may not always be what you had hoped for or wanted, but you can separate the wheat from the chaff and keep whatever you feel is relevant and important. Interaction with others will also provide you with specific events and incidents to remember, during which you may have shown qualities of kindness, caring and understanding. This will give you something concrete with which to fortify your sense of self-worth whenever you feel you are of no value.

The importance of being accountable for your own actions was emphasized earlier in the book, and it still applies, but it should be possible to do this as part of a human network in which you share with others and listen as they share with you.

The concept of sharing may make you uneasy if, perhaps from past experience, you are wary of letting down barriers in case you get hurt. You may have felt, or still feel, the heartache which comes with the end of an important relationship, and decide that it is safer to retreat into a protective shell than to risk being hurt all over again. Or the matter may be less cut and dried. You may feel caught in a dilemma of longing for closeness on the one hand, and being afraid of it on the other.

There can be no doubt that opening up to others is a risky

undertaking, since the response is unpredictable. At the end of the day it is for each individual to decide whether or not to take this risk, but since reaching out is such a basic human impulse, based on need, the cost to those who fight against it can be high, particularly if they suffer from bulimia. Such people probably remain isolated and therefore vulnerable to the fleeting comfort of binge-eating, and its aftermath of anxiety, poor self-esteem, and depression.

Helpful hints

1. Try to accept your need of others and to communicate. Aim to build a few trusting relationships. However unlovable or unworthy you think you are, you are probably not the best judge of yourself. As with all of us, some will like you and others will not. Other people should, however, have the opportunity of finding out for themsevles what they think of you.

2. Go out and join people, rather than shutting yourself away and becoming self-absorbed. Decide on something you would like to do and use it as an incentive to meet people you have something in common with. Find out about social events, mother and toddler groups, evening classes, gardening clubs and so forth from libraries, shop windows, and newspapers.

3. Aim to be with people who will enable you to get your anxieties about food, eating and weight into perspective.

   I cut down my exposure to people who were very diet conscious – always skipping lunch and jumping on and off scales. It was necessary for me to do this. I'm so sensitive about the subject myself and knew I would be easily persuaded to try the latest fad diet or fitness craze.

4. Try to cultivate one or two close women friends with whom you can have some 'girl talk'. It helps to know there are others who have to put up with monthly miseries, difficult partners, pushy parents or bawling babies.

5. Keep close to family and friends. Whether they seek solace in drugs, alcohol or bulimia, people who do well

when it comes to kicking the habit are invariably those with supportive backgrounds. So do not shut out the important people in your life. They are best able to give you the immediate and the long-term support you need. There will probably be times when your aims and ideas run counter to theirs, but it will be easier for them to try to meet you half way if you keep them in the picture. Be patient with them, and remember that any changes you intend to make in your lifestyle will affect them too, and they may need time to adjust.

Take the time and trouble to explain to them, as best you can, why food plays such an important role in your life, and ways in which they can contribute to your recovery.

6. Try not to link your sense of self-worth to the opinions of others. It is natural to want approval, but you will never be able to please everyone, and no matter how consistently you behave, people will always judge you differently. Remember, too, that a person's critiscism or disapproval of you may not be valid. It may stem from irrational thinking, jealousy or resentment, in which case they are the ones who need a change of heart.

7. Try not to pick holes in yourself. Remember that you are acceptable as a person, and whatever your problems, you have qualities which can be used and appreciated.

If you are still not convinced, build up your sense of self-worth by making a list of (a) five things that you like about yourself; (b) five areas of life that you are interested in; (c) five things that you have done in the past which you think are interesting and/or worthwhile. Stick your list where you can see it regularly, such as by your bedside table, in your bag, by the kitchen sink or your bedroom mirror. It will help to remind you that life is not so bad.

21.

VALUING YOUR HEALTH

Sufferers from bulimia are prone to ill-effects of the behaviour, and unfortunately, many lose sight of the importance of taking care of their bodies in a general sense. They can become so preoccupied with trying to look attractively slim that they completely overlook the deterioration in their physical appearance.

> With every ounce I lost I was convinced I was becoming more attractive. I wanted to be willowy – to have that faint look of the lost child about me. Instead I ended up looking a mess, with my swollen face, my bloodshot eyes and my rotting teeth. I felt wretched almost all of the time and became a nightmare to live with.

Advice is given below about how best to take care of yourself to minimize the detrimental effects of bulimia.

Weaning off laxatives and/or diuretics
Work out some sort of fixed withdrawal plan. If you have abused laxatives heavily and over a long period of time, aim to phase them out gradually. This will help to lessen the distressing effects of rebound water retention.

Fight the temptation to take laxatives or diuretics to get rid of water retention if and when it occurs. This will only perpetuate your dependency on them for making you feel slim, and increase the risk of kidney damage.

Rebound constipation
To relieve rebound constipation and restore normal bowel function, take plenty of fluid, a reasonable amount of roughage, and exercise. Bulking agents such as Normacol or Fibrogel may be helpful in the short term. These work

by absorbing water into the bowel and increasing the bulk of the motions without causing irritation to the colon in the way that laxatives such as senna and cascara do. If you think that you need a bulking agent, discuss the matter with your doctor beforehand.

Potassium supplements

Your doctor may suggest you take potassium supplements in the form of tablets if your blood potassium levels are very low. This mineral can also be found in the following list of foods: bananas and tomatoes (particularly rich sources), jacket potatoes, leafy vegetables, peaches, plums, peas, beans and lentils.

Remember, however, that potassium supplements in any form will be ineffective unless they are fully digested.

Care of your teeth

Many sufferers make the mistake of scrubbing their teeth straight after being sick. This in fact damages the surface crystals on the enamel layer of the teeth. Dentists who specialize in problems related to enamel erosion advise that, after being sick, you rinse your mouth out thoroughly with water or a sodium bicarbonate mouthwash, and then wait several hours before having anything acidic, such as fruit or fizzy drinks, and especially before brushing your teeth. In conjunction with saliva, this treatment has a neutralizing effect on the stomach acid which seeps into the surface enamel after vomiting. If you clean your teeth whilst they are in this sensitive state, abrasive properties in toothpaste etch the enamel still further, so that over the years it is progressively worn away.

If you feel compelled to brush your teeth after being sick, avoid using toothpaste, particularly smokers' toothpaste. Just use a brush dipped in water.

Recent research has also shown that you can minimize the detrimental effects of acidity on dental enamel by eating cheese or drinking milk, but obviously, if eating these foods is likely to propel you into a panic binge, then just settle for rinsing out your mouth with water.

It is a good idea to tell your dentist about your eating problem. It saves having to invent stories to account for the deterioration or fragile state of your teeth.

Go for regular check-ups at least every six months, and more often if your gums bleed a lot. This is particularly important if you have a high frequency of bingeing and vomiting.

Controlling your weight

If you are genuinely overweight for your height and age you will probably be tempted to lose it at some stage. Beware of 'wonder diets' and drugs. Most of them have no nutritional back-up and do nothing to re-educate your eating habits. Remember, there are no short cuts to long-term weight loss. The best way to lose weight is to follow a gradual and properly balanced diet of no less than 1,000 calories a day. Total fasting and 'protein' liquid diets can also be harmful, expensive and a waste of effort. Furthermore, unless you stick to a varied and nutritionally balanced daily intake of food, it is unlikely that you will ever make any real progress towards getting better.

A helpful book to read is *The A–Z of Slimming* by Professor John Yudkin (Coronet, 1981). In it he scotches many of the myths of the slimming industry and offers a lot of down-to-earth advice.

Exercising ... in moderation

There is no need to become a keep-fit fanatic, as many bulimia sufferers do, but a reasonable amount of exercise will do you a lot of good. Many people find that taking some form of exercise helps them to control a tendency to smoke, eat or drink too much. Apart from helping them to feel physically fitter, exercise provides them with a healthy outlet for pent-up aggressions and frustrations, thereby improving their sense of mental well-being. This in turn boosts their self-confidence, reduces their vulnerability to stress, and improves relationships. Furthermore, swimming, cycling, keep-fit classes and raquet games are all forms of exercise which can improve your social life, as well as helping you to control your weight.

Bulimia and contraception

The pill is not a reliable method of contraception for bulimia sufferers because it has to be taken regularly to be effective. Sickness and diarrhoea can make it pass out of the body before it has been absorbed. If this happens, you are not protected against becoming pregnant, and you may well not realize the fact.

If you are on the pill, try to take it at a time of the day when you know you are unlikely to binge and purge, and allow several hours to digest it properly. If you are sick a lot, abuse laxatives, have a tendency to absent-mindedness or have a disorganized lifestyle, you should probably think about an alternative method of contraception. Have a chat to your doctor or family planning clinic about this.

Anyone who experiences wide fluctuations in their size and weight and who is using, or planning to use, the cap or diaphragm as a method of contraception, should also be aware that the size and shape of the vagina can alter if you lose or gain about 10 pounds. To be effective the cap needs to fit snugly over the neck of the womb and if your internal measurements have altered it may slip out of place. If you do decide to use the cap, and are prone to significant weight changes, remember to go to your doctor or family planning clinic for regular check-ups.

Pregnancy

Studies have shown that pregnancy can be associated with a decrease in bulimic behaviour, but this appears to diminish during the first year after childbirth, and few women completely recover. A variety of factors may contribute to this transient improvement including concern for the developing child, hormonal changes and increased attention from others. Release from concern about body image because of an expected weight gain may be another reason.

There is no scientific evidence as yet to show that bingeing and vomiting have any detrimental effects on the babies of sufferers, and some women have given birth to perfectly normal and healthy babies whilst in the throes of quite severe bulimia. Many health care workers stress the importance of a balanced diet during pregnancy, however, because they believe that poor nutrition affects a baby's birthweight and growth potential. Their views sometimes cause consternation amongst sufferers who for one reason or another are unable to make a clean break from their behaviour even when they become pregnant, and who therefore fear that their babies will be physically or mentally retarded. The emotional strain of worrying may be severe enough to drive them into a more intense cycle of bingeing/purging in an effort to blot out their apprehensions. There is another school of thought, however, which believes that the effect of diet on a baby's development and survival is exaggerated. Sufferers who are pregnant and anxious about the consequences of their behaviour on their unborn child may be interested in the views expressed in *Pregnancy* by Gordon Bourne, an obstetrician and gynaecologist (Pan, revised edition 1984). He writes:

> It is difficult to influence the birthweight of a baby by diet during pregnancy. The baby is a parasite and behaves as one. It will extract from the maternal circulation its exact and complete requirements regardless of the mother's condition.

He gives iron and calcium as examples of minerals which the baby will remove from the mother in order to have healthy blood and to develop normal bones. Thus it is likely to be the mother's rather than the baby's health which suffers as a result of mineral deficiencies, and she will need to take supplements in order to avoid becoming anaemic and/or developing softened bones.

Despite these views, it is obviously better to play safe and try to overcome bulimia before becoming pregnant. Your baby may not suffer nutritional deficiencies but will still be at risk if you experience dizzy spells, blackouts and poor co-ordination after being sick. Driving a car, crossing roads, or going up or down stairs and escalators, can be hazardous under these conditions. Severe attacks of gastro-enteritis (similar to the effects of a liberal dose of laxatives) and extremes of physical activity (think of the physical force involved in vomiting) have been linked with miscarriage, as have accidents such as falling down stairs or being in a car crash. Premature labour has also been associated with emotional or physical shock, and babies born several weeks early may develop complications. Some premature babies are unable to suck, breathe, or keep themselves warm enough.

Intensified guilt may be another problem which affects sufferers who are pregnant. It is common for women to feel guilt over complications which may arise during the development or birth of their baby, even if they are in no way responsible. Women with bulimia are particularly prone to such self-reproach because they often believe that their behaviour is at the root of the trouble.

> I'd had a long labour and my contractions became too weak to push the baby out. The doctors decided to speed things up with a forceps delivery because the baby was getting tired. Whilst all this was going on I began thinking that the problem was related to my chaotic eating habits, and that it might also be some sort of divine punishment intended to make me care for myself and my baby rather better than I had been. After the birth, when Gemma was brought to me with red marks on her face, the feeling that everything was my fault was reinforced. Despite being reassured that the marks were temporary, and the result of being delivered by forceps, I kept thinking, 'Trust them to find a rational explanation. If only they knew. I'm to blame. She must have got battered and bruised when she was inside me and I was bingeing and vomiting throughout the day.' I heaped blame on myself for weeks.

Nagging guilt may ultimately lead to feelings of inadequacy, whereby sufferers lose confidence in their ability to care for and cope with the demands of a baby, and the mother/baby relationship becomes fraught with tension.

Some sufferers are doubly unfortunate in that as well as their Bulimia they are victims of alcohol and/or drug addiction. As with women who do not have Bulimia, it is vital that they stop their alcohol and/or drug intake as well as endeavouring to keep their Bulimia under control. A baby will receive its blood supply from yours whilst it is in your womb. If drugs and/or alcohol are in your bloodstream, the baby gets a dose as well. No one knows exactly how much you can drink without risk to your baby, but recent research shows that 'drinking mothers' sometimes give birth to babies with a group of features known as 'the alcohol foetal syndrome'. They may have malformed heads, be slow to develop physically and suffer mental defects. Drugs may be an additional source of potential harm to your developing baby. It may be physically perfect but become addicted whilst in your womb, and experience distressing withdrawal effects after it has been born.

Apart from the potential physical risks to your baby,

there are the possible emotional effects on your offspring to consider. Bulimia can have far-reaching and quite devastating effects on relationships in general, including those with your children. Mothers who are addicted to drugs, alcohol or binge-eating may not give the family the attention and care that it needs. Also, children can be very perceptive and quick to pick up on their mother's anxieties. As a result they can come to feel insecure themselves, and this may be reflected in behavioural problems such as running away from school or home, shoplifting or bedwetting. No studies have been carried out into the emotional impact on the children of bulimia sufferers, but the thought that there could be harmful consequences may provide you with a powerful incentive to give it up.

Having a drink .... now and then

Alcohol has been an integral part of all cultures for thousands of years and the evidence is that consumption has increased markedly in all countries over the past 30 years.[1] In present times there are many occasions when alcohol is consumed. For many people alcohol is a pleasant aid to relaxation, for others, however, consumption of alcohol goes beyond this to become an integral part of their life, tending both to damage it and to assume a position whereby they cannot continue without it. Where to draw the line between taking an acceptable amount of alcohol and being overtaken by it is difficult to determine. Personal variation in alcohol tolerance is considerable both between individuals and indeed between men and women. As a general guide your alcohol consumption may be considered excessive when it impinges on your life in ways which are outlined below.

During the last three months

Have you woken up and been unable to
remember some of the things you had
done while drinking the previous night?   Yes   No

[1] Plant M.A. Drinking and Problem Drinking 1982 (Junction Books)

Have you been in arguments with your family or friends because of your drinking?	Yes	No
Have you found that your hands were shaking in the morning after drinking in the previous evening?	Yes	No
Have you felt ashamed or guilty about your drinking?	Yes	No
Has your work suffered in any way because of drinking?	Yes	No
Have you found yourself neglecting any of your responsibilities because of drinking?	Yes	No
Have you had a drink first thing in the morning to steady your nerves or to get rid of a hangover?	Yes	No
Has there been any occasion when you felt unable to stop drinking?	Yes	No
Have you feared that you were becoming dependent on alcohol?	Yes	No
Have you needed a drink to face certain situations or problems?	Yes	No
Have you had financial difficulties because of drink?	Yes	No
Have you given up hobbies, sports or other interests and spent more time drinking instead?	Yes	No
Have you concealed the amount you drink from those close to you?	Yes	No
Have you been drunk for several days running?	Yes	No
Have you been violent after drinking?	Yes	No
Have you been arrested for drunkenness?	Yes	No

If you have answered 'Yes' to any of these questions, drink is causing you problems and you do have a reason for cutting down.

Taken from *So You Want to Cut down Your Drinking?* Scottish Health Education Group.

In any event, current advice from The Health Education Council in their free booklet 'That's The Limit' recommend that men should not exceed about 10 pints of beer, equivalent to roughly 3 bottles of wine, and women not more than about 7 pints of beer, or two bottles of wine, per week. The harmful effects of alcohol intoxication are listed in it on page 56 under the heading 'Harmful effects of drug stimulants and alcohol abuse'. For those who feel that their alcohol consumption is excessive there is a variety of helpful literature which outlines practical strategies for tackling this problem and these are listed in the bibliography.

If you are someone who binge eats and binge drinks, try to tackle both problems at the same time so that you do not end up substituting one method of coping with life's problems for another.

In addition to the available literature, there are a number of organisations which offer specialist help to anyone who feels they need it. Their names and addresses are listed in the back of the book.

Dealing with drugs

Seek medical help if you have been abusing amphetamines. Sudden withdrawal can lead to distressing symptoms, and your doctor may be able to help you formulate a weaning plan which will not be too psychologically or physically traumatic. At present there is no blueprint for curing drug addiction of any sort. If your doctor thinks you need long-term support, he may refer you to a hospital-based specialist (where you will probably attend as an outpatient) or suggest that you apply to an agency with an interest in the treatment and rehabilitation of people who abuse drugs. Group techniques are often used by these agencies, and the majority have a counselling service for relatives and friends as well as the drug abusers themselves. The address of SCODA, a national drugs information and advisory service is included in the list of addresses at the back of the book.

22.

MAKING HEADWAY

It will probably be clear by now that there are no instant solutions or formulae for overcoming bulimia. As a result you may be wondering if you will ever really be free of it. A question for you to think about is what recovery means to you personally. You may take the view that you must stop bingeing completely in order to consider yourself 'cured'. This is an approach adopted by many alcoholics and drug abusers, but it is not terribly realistic for bulimia sufferers. Like everyone else, you have to eat to live, and along with many 'normal' eaters you will probably always remain vulnerable to 'comfort eating' during moments of stress, boredom, depression and so on. A lot will also depend on how you define a binge, and whether you are able to see a session of over-eating for what it is, rather than a relapse, or a failure to succeed in what you set out to do. Again, the subject of goal-keeping crops up, and the importance of keeping your goals realistic extends to your hopes for recovery. An important step forward for many is an ability to keep a sense of proportion about setbacks. This comes with the realization that they are not (and indeed never have been) in the power of some terrible outside force that is leading them down a path of self-destruction. They feel confident that they are in control of what they do, as opposed to feeling 'driven', and are no longer slaves to their food cravings.

Recovery can therefore mean different things to different individuals, and the time it takes to reach a stage of feeling in control or cured will also vary from person to person. Apart from stabilizing your eating there will be other problems to face up to and deal with. Some of these will have arisen as a consequence of your bulimia, and will therefore resolve themselves at the same time that your eating difficulties subside. Others will remain as 'unfinished business' in one form or another; perhaps you need to adjust to an earlier loss, or to express yourself more honestly instead of always feeling that you have to curb your true personality, or to simply accept yourself and your limitations. It is quite fitting that overcoming bulimia has been described as something of a learning and restorative process, in which you literally begin to piece yourself together. In doing so, you steadily discover all sorts of things about yourself, what you feel and do, and how you relate to other people, as you grow out of your bulimia. For many, this process is slow and uneven. There are times when it is painful and therefore difficult to keep up the necessary motivation to change, but what really matters is that deep down you want it to happen. This means being prepared to come to terms with yourself, to give up frustrated desires to be like someone else and allowing others to see you for what you really are. Being able to do this, in addition to establishing a relaxed attitude towards food, brings about a great sense of liberation, as well as an awakening of all your senses. Suddenly you can appreciate the little things in life – a morning mist, a warm smile, dancing autumn leaves, someone's carefree laughter – which you probably never had the time, energy or inclination to notice whilst you were in the throes of your bulimia, and which make you aware of the joy and gladness that is to be found in truly living.

As you work towards your goals, however, it is important that you respect your own pace. The changes which you are striving for will not come about in a flash of inspiration, or through pills, potions or anyone else's words of wisdom. Realizing this is essential and once you have accepted that the responsibility and potential for change lie with you, tension will flow out of your life because you are no longer looking to others to provide you with the answers. The way forward will become increasingly clear and with a bit of imagination and a lot of courage, commitment, honesty and determination, you too, in the words of a former sufferer, 'can begin to get your life back'.

USEFUL ADDRESSES

When writing to any of the organizations listed below, it is a good idea to enclose a stamped addressed envelope to ensure a prompt reply.

The Eating Disorders Association
(formerly Anorexic Aid and Anorexic Family Aid)
Sackville Place
44–48 Magdalen Street
Norwich
Norfolk NR3 1JU
Tel: (0603) 621414

The Eating Disorders Association offers information and understanding through telephone help-lines, guidelines, newsletters and a national network of self-help groups for anorexic and bulimic sufferers and their families.

The Women's Therapy Centre
6–9 Manor Gardens
London N7 6LA
Tel: 071–263 6200
(Calls are answered between 2–4.30 p.m. weekdays.)

Offers feminist psychotherapy to women. Individual and group therapy. Workshops on eating disorders.

The Scottish Centre for Eating Disorders
3 Sciennes Road
Edinburgh EH9 1LE
Tel: (031) 668 3051

The Maisner Centre for Eating Disorders
P.O. Box 464
Hove
East Sussex BN3 2BN
Tel: (0273) 729818 or 29334

The British Association of Psychotherapists
37 Mapesbury Road
London NW2 4HJ
Tel: 081–452 9823

This is a registered charity and professional body for psychotherapists. Write to the Secretary for details of practitioners in your area.

SCODA (Standing Conference on Drug Abuse)
1–4 Hatton Place
Hatton Garden
London EC1N 8ND
Tel: 071–430 2341

The national co-ordinating body for the drugs field. Help
and advice is available on all aspects of drug abuse. A regularly updated guide to services in the UK for people with
drug problems is also available.

ADFAM NATIONAL
First Floor
Chapel House
18 Hatton Place
London EC1N 8ND
Tel: 071–405 3923

Runs the national helpline for the families and friends of
drug users. Counselling, friendship, information about
drugs and details of family support projects within the UK
are available 10 a.m.–5 p.m. Mondays to Fridays. An
answerphone giving an emergency number operates at
other times.

Alcoholics Anonymous
General Service Office
4th Floor, P.O. Box 1
Stonebow House
Stonebow
York YO1 2NJ
Tel: (0904) 644026

This organization helps anyone with a drink problem who wants to overcome it. Information about groups throughout the UK, including times and places of meetings can be obtained from this office.

Al-Anon Family Groups (UK and Eire)
61 Great Dover Street
London SE1 4YF
Tel: 071–403 0888

A similar organization to Alcoholics Anonymous. It helps the families and friends of problem drinkers. Information about meetings can be obtained from the London headquarters.

Alateen
For young people (aged 12–20) whose lives have been affected by someone else's drinking. Contact them through Al-Anon.

The National Osteoporosis Society
P.O. Box 10
Radstock
Bath BA3 3YB
Tel: (0761) 432472
Helpline: (0761) 431594

Support and advice on the causes, treatment and prevention of osteoporosis.

The Portia Trust
Portia Centre
Workspace
Maryport
Cumbria CA15 8NF
Tel: (0900) 812114 (day)
      (06973) 51820 (any other time)

The Portia Trust is a national charity which campaigns for
changes in the law affecting women's rights. It also provides help, advice and friendship to anyone who is in trouble with the law as a result of mental illness, nervous
breakdown and poverty. Those who work at the trust are
not concerned with helping deliberate criminals but they
are anxious to support anyone who becomes severely distressed as a result of shop-lifting allegations, for example,
including people who have an underlying depressive or
mental illness that may have caused them to steal.

FURTHER READING

Eating Disorders

Suzanne Abraham and Derek Llewellyn-Jones, *Eating Disorders: The Facts* (Oxford University Press, 1984).

Marlene Boskind-White, *Bulimarexia: The Binge/Purge Cycle*, (W.W. Norton, 1984).

Hilde Bruch, *Eating Disorders: Obesity, Anorexia Nervosa and the Person Within*, (Routledge and Kegan Paul 1974).

Peter J. Dally and Joan Gomez, *Obesity and Anorexia Nervosa: A Question of Shape*, (Faber and Faber, 1980). Written by two psychiatrists experienced in dealing with people suffering from eating disorders.

Peter Lambley, *How to Survive Anorexia (A guide to Anorexia and Bulimia)*, (Frederick Muller, 1983).

Marilyn Lawrence, *The Anorexic Experience*, (The Women's Press Handbook Series, 1984).

Paulette Maisner, *The Food Trap*, (Allen & Unwin).

Joy Melville, *ABC of Eating*, (Sheldon Press, 1983).

Susie Orbach, *Fat is a Feminist Issue 1 and 2,* (Hamlyn Paperbacks, 1978, 1982), Including self-help tapes.

Louis Roche, *Glutton for Punishment*, (Pan, 1984).
A personal account of her experience of bulimia.

Reducing Stress

Leon Chaitow, *Relaxation and Meditation Techniques*, (Thorsons, 1983).
Meditation, visualization and breathing techniques, as well as sound advice on nutrition and exercise, are included in this natural relaxation system which will help you cope more easily with stress and its related symptoms.

Consumer's Association, *Living With Stress*, (1982).
Looks at a wide range of life experiences which cause stress, explains the signs and symptoms of stress and stress-related diseases, and contains a comprehensive chapter on methods of self-help for reducing stress in our lives.

Jane Madders, *Stress and Relaxation*, (Martin Dunitz, 1980).
This book explains the causes of stress, how to recognize it and what we can do to counteract the ill-effects which too much stress has on our lives. Photographs of people demonstrating relaxation techniques make this book particularly easy to follow.

Dr Eric Trimmer, *The 10-Day Relaxation Plan*, (Piatkus Books, 1984).
A well-illustrated self-help book containing three ten-day schemes to suit different age groups and circumstances. The causes of stress and how it effects us are examined, and alternative means of dealing with stress-related illnesses are also covered.

Gender Role Conditioning

Carol Adams and Rae Laurikietis, *The Gender Trap*, (Virage, 1976).
There are three books in this series, Book 3 is of particular interest to people with eating disorders. It deals with the messages and images which we receive from language, humour and the media and their effects on both sexes.

Joyce Nicholson, *What Society Does To Girls*, (Virago, 1980).
Explains how and why gender role conditioning occurs, and suggests ways in which the status of women in society might be improved.

Dealing with Depression
Jack Dominion, *Depression*, (Fontana, 1976).
Examines the causes of depression, the classification of different types of depression, how common it is, who it may affect, how to manage it, and current available forms of treatment.

Dr John Rush, *Beating Depression*, (Century Publishing, 1983).
Offers clear advice and up to date information on current methods of treating depression (including the Cognitive Theory).

Dr Caroline Shreeve, *Depression*, (Thorsons, 1984).
Explains depressive illness, its causes and standard forms of therapy which are currently available. Also contains a personalized programme to help sufferers learn to cope with stress and explains the importance of developing a positive outlook on life.

Dr Andrew Stanway, *Overcoming Depression*, (Hamlyn, 1981).
Offers sympathetic advice for sufferers and their families.

Vivienne Welburn, *Postnatal Depression*, (Fontana, 1980).
A book which will provide comfort and reassurance to anyone experiencing, or who has experienced, 'baby blues'. Examines the nature of postnatal depression and social, physical, and psychological reasons why it occurs. The book is based on interviews with many mothers.

Premenstrual Syndrome
Dr Michael Brush, *Understanding Pre-Menstrual Tension*, (Pan, 1984).
Explains how to recognize symptoms, why they arise and the treatment available, either from doctors, self-help or over-the-counter medicine.

Dr Caroline Shreeve, *The Premenstrual Syndrome: The Curse that Can be Cured*, (Thorsons, 1983).
Explains what the premenstrual syndrome is, its causes, effects, current available treatment and what women can do to help themselves to alleviate the symptoms.

Positive Thinking and Assertiveness

Norman Vincent Peale, *The Power of Positive Thinking*, (World's Work, 1953).
Explains how cultivating a positive attitude of mind can help you to throw off despondency about life and improve you emotional and physical well-being.

Ann Dickson, *A Woman In Your Own Right*, (Quartet, 1982).
Looks at the anger and frustrations which can arise from compliance with traditional ideas about a woman's role. Aimed at helping readers to put aside the need for approval, enabling them to make their own decisions.

Self-Help

Sheila Ernst and Lucy Goodison, *In Our Own Hands*, (The Women's Press, 1981).
Useful for anyone interested in setting up or participating in a self-help group. Describes many therapy approaches and contains practical advice.

Oliver Gillie, Angela Price, and Sharon Robinson, *The Sunday Times Self-Help Directory*, (Granada, 1982).
Whatever your problems or needs this excellent book lists a vast number of self-help organizations' which will provide you with information, advice and support. It is available from public libraries and is updated regularly.

Alternative Medicine

Dr Andrew Stanway, *Alternative Medicine*, (Pelican Books, 1979).
Anyone considering a branch of alternative medicine for dealing with their bulimia will find this book helpful when selecting a therapy that suits them. It provides information on thirty two therapies, including aromatherapy, hydrotherapy, colour therapy and hypnosis.

Women's Health

Angela Phillips and Jill Rakusen, *Our Bodies Ourselves*, (Penguin, 1978).
An excellent book on female biology, contraception, sexuality and other aspects of women's health. Includes accounts of personal experiences.

Problem Drinking

J. Chick and J. Chick, *Drinking Problems: information and advice for the individual, family and friends* (Churchill Livingstone, 1984).

M. Grant, *Same Again: a guide to safer drinking,* (Penguin, 1984).

Health Education Council, *That's The Limit: a guide to sensible drinking,* (1983).

M.A. Plant, *Drinking and Problem Drinking*, (Junction Books, 1982).

I. Robertson and N. Heather, *So you want to cut down your drinking: a self-help guide to sensible drinking,* (Scottish Health Education Group, 1984).

Report by Special Committee of The Royal College of Psychiatrists, *Alcohol and Alcoholism*, (Tavistock Publications, 1979).
Explains the nature and causes of harmful drinking, its effects, and current methods of treating alcoholism, and outlines necessary steps for overcoming alcohol dependence.

Cooking and Nutrition

Delia Smith, *One is Fun!* (Hodder and Stoughton, 1981).
There are many books on the subject of health foods and diet. Although these contain dietary advice, the approach which deals with 'good' and 'bad' foods is probably unhelpful for those people who have pre-existing worries about food. This book however avoids this form of classification and gives well balanced and easy to prepare recipes for people who are eating alone. Many people

cannot be bothered to cook just for themselves, and for bulimia victims this can lead to trouble in the form of bingeing on convenience foods. *One is Fun!* demonstrates that cooking for yourself need not involve too much time, effort or expense, and that it can be enjoyable. This book is also particularly helpful for people who are unclear as to what constitutes a normal helping for a single person, and the recipes can be adapted for four people.

Ministry of Agriculture and Food, *Manual of Nutrition*, (Her Majesty's Stationery Office, revised edition 1993). A comprehensive guide to all aspects of nutrition.

INDEX

Of related interest . . .

CONSUMING PASSIONS

What to Do When Food Rules Your Life

Paulette Maisner
with Rosemary Turner

Why is it that some people eat quite simply for health and pleasure, while for many others the world of food becomes a dark and secret nightmare?

Paulette Maisner has spent many years counselling people who are excessively worried about their weight. Her highly successful eating plan has saved hundreds of chronic dieters from the chaos of yo-yo dieting and obsessive calorie counting or the extremes of bulimia and anorexia.

Drawing on her own experience, using self-help questionnaires and personal stories, Paulette's tough but successful approach will help you to recognize when food is beginning to rule your life and learn how to understand and control it.

This practical and realistic book will help you to:

- overcome eating problems
- understand your hunger cycles
- recognize your trigger foods
- control your blood sugar levels
- improve your self-esteem
- get control of your moods – and your life

CONSUMING PASSIONS	0 7225 2703 9	£7.99	☐
OBSESSIVE COMPULSIVE DISORDER	0 7225 2912 0	£6.99	☐
COMING OFF TRANQUILLIZERS AND SLEEPING PILLS	0 7225 2398 X	£5.99	☐
SUPER-POTENCY	0 7225 2841 8	£7.99	☐
OVERCOME INCONTINENCE	0 7225 2937 6	£5.99	☐
TINNITUS	0 7225 2940 6	£5.99	☐
BACK PAIN	0 7225 2961 9	£5.99	☐
BEAT PSORIASIS	0 7225 2586 9	£7.99	☐

All these books are available from your local bookseller or can be ordered direct from the publishers.

To order direct just tick the titles you want and fill in the form below:

Name: _____

Address: _____

_____

_____ Postcode: _____

Send to: Thorsons Mail Order, Dept 3, HarperCollins*Publishers*, Westerhill Road, Bishopbriggs, Glasgow G64 2QT.
Please enclose a cheque or postal order or your authority to debit your Visa/Access account —

Credit card no: _____

Expiry date: _____

Signature: _____

— to the value of the cover price plus:
UK & BFPO: Add £1.00 for the first book and 25p for each additional book ordered.
Overseas orders including Eire: Please add £2.95 service charge. Books will be sent by surface mail but quotes for airmail despatches will be given on request.

24 HOUR TELEPHONE ORDERING SERVICE FOR ACCESS/VISA CARDHOLDERS — TEL: **041 772 2281.**